AIDS
—What Every Student Needs to Know

Spencer A. Rathus, Ph.D.
St. John's University

Susan Boughn, R.N., Ed.D.
Trenton State College

Harcourt Brace Jovanovich College Publishers

Fort Worth · Philadelphia · San Diego
New York · Orlando · Austin · San Antonio
Toronto · Montreal · London · Sydney · Tokyo

Publisher	Ted Buchholz
Acquisitions Editor	Eve Howard
Developmental Editor	John Haley
Project Editor	Erica Lazerow
Production Manager	Thomas Urquhart
Cover Design	John Ritland
Cover Photo Researcher	Lois Fichner-Rathus

ISBN: 0-15-500724-6

Address Editorial Correspondence To: 301 Commerce Street, Suite 3700
Fort Worth TX 76102

Address Orders To: 6277 Sea Harbor Drive
Orlando FL 32887
1-800-782-4479, or 1-800-433-0001 (in Florida)

Printed in the United States of America.

3 4 5 6 7 8 9 0 1 2 095 9 8 7 6 5 4 3 2

Contents

Preface v

Chapter 1 TESTING YOUR AIDS AWARENESS 1

The AIDS Awareness Inventory 3 · Answers to the AIDS Awareness Inventory 4

Chapter 2 AIDS—THE FIRST DECADE 10

AIDS—The First Decade: A Time Line 11

Chapter 3 AIDS AND THE IMMUNE SYSTEM 23

Ways in Which the Body Defends Itself Against Disease 23 · The Immune System 25 · Human Immunodeficiency Virus (H.I.V.) and the Immune System 25 · Course of H.I.V. Infection and AIDS 27 · Indicator and Opportunistic Diseases 28 · Women and AIDS 28 · Children and AIDS 32 · Adjustment of People with H.I.V. Infections and AIDS 32

Chapter 4 TRANSMISSION, DIAGNOSIS, AND TREATMENT

Transmission of H.I.V. 34 · Diagnosis 42 · Treatment 45

Chapter 5 OTHER SEXUALLY TRANSMITTED DISEASES 47

STDs Caused by Bacteria 48 · Vaginitis 57 · STDs Caused by Viruses 59 · STDs Caused by Parasites 62

Chapter 6 PREVENTION 63

Abstinence—What Is It? 64 · A Lifelong Monogamous Relationship—How Do You Get There from Here? 65 · The Truth about 'Safe Sex'—It's Really Safer Sex 66 · Resisting Sexual Pressure: What It Is, What to Do 71

Notes 82

Bibliography 83

Dedication

*To Richard, childhood friend, best man
at my wedding, and living with AIDS.*
                              –Susan Boughn

A Note To Readers:

This book is as up-to-date as we can make it, but there is an almost continuous flow of new information about H.I.V. infection and AIDS. The U.S. government Centers for Disease Control has established a toll-free hotline to answer your questions. You need not identify yourself when you call. You can find more information, for example, on the symptoms of AIDS, diagnostic methods, and treatment. The number is:

AIDS Toll-Free Hotline Number: 1-800-342-AIDS

If you want to ask your questions and receive your answers *en español*, dial

AIDS/SIDA Toll-Free Hotline Number: 1-800-344-SIDA

Preface

This is the book we did not want to have to write. After it was written, we hoped that a medical breakthrough would make it obsolete before it ever reached your hands. As health professionals and teachers, however, we had no choice but to write it. Nor has the long-sought medical breakthrough occurred. Unfortunately, or fortunately—depending on your point of view—the book has thus remained timely.

Our purpose in writing is simple: to save lives. Most college students are in their late teens or early twenties, and that is a time of life when one can feel invulnerable to illness. Would that it were so! During the years of early adulthood sexual impulses can be overwhelming, drinking can be heavy, and fears of social rejection can be powerful. The personal myth of invulnerability in combination with these other forces can put students at risk for auto accidents, unwanted pregnancies, and—the focus of our book—being infected with the AIDS virus and microorganisms that give rise to other sexually transmitted diseases.

You may have heard horrible things about H.I.V. infection and AIDS, and you may be wondering whether they are true. We cannot comment on what you have heard from other sources, but we promise you that we won't try to sell you any phony horror stories in order to get you to change your behavior. The *true* story, sad to say, is grave enough.

Although there is good reason to fear AIDS, there is also some good news: AIDS is preventable. That is what this book is all about—helping you find ways of preventing AIDS that are compatible with your own values.

This book, as mentioned in Chapter 1, could be considered R-rated. It contains sex and it contains nudity—enough sex and nudity for us to tell our story. It does *not* contain violence, however. Our goal is to help you prevent doing violence to yourself and to the people whom you care about.

About the Authors

Spencer A. Rathus, Ph.D., is a psychologist on the faculty at St. John's University. His areas of interest include health psychology, sexual behavior, psychological assessment, and methods of therapy. Dr. Rathus's articles appear in professional journals, including *Behavior Therapy*, *Journal of Clinical Psychology*, *Behaviour Research and Therapy*, *Journal of Behavior Therapy and Experimental Psychiatry*, *Adolescence*, and *Criminology*. Other books by Dr. Rathus include *Psychology*, *Adjustment and Growth*, *Essentials of Psychology*, *Thinking and Writing About Psychology*, *Abnormal Psychology*, *Making the Most of College*, and *Human Sexuality in a World of Diversity*.

Susan Boughn, R.N., Ed.D., is associate professor of nursing at Trenton State College. She conducts research and publishes in professional journals such as *Nursing and Health Care* and *The Journal of Nursing Education*. She lectures nationally and internationally—in settings as diverse as California and the People's Republic of China. Dr. Boughn's areas of interest include infectious diseases, maternal child health, contraceptive science, public health nursing, and health issues that are specific to women. A special concern of Dr. Boughn is the empowering of women to obtain adequate health care.

Acknowledgments

We wish to thank our professional colleagues who have painstakingly read over this manuscript to ensure that it would be accurate. We also wish to express our gratitude to Bill Barnett, Eve Howard, Michael Alread, John Haley, and the other fine publishing professionals at Harcourt Brace Jovanovich for their faith in this book and in us.

1 Testing Your AIDS Awareness

●*AIDS.* In 1990, *The New England Journal of Medicine* reports that two in every thousand college students are infected with H.I.V., the microscopic organism that causes AIDS.[1]

●*AIDS.* In 1991, the World Health Organization estimates that 10 million people around the world are infected with H.I.V.[2]

●*AIDS.* In 1992, 6 of the 197 students enrolled at Rivercrest High School in Bogata, Texas, are reported to be infected with H.I.V. A resident of this rural town remarks on Bogata's new place in the limelight: 'Bogata is going to be identified with AIDS forever, and maybe the only good part is that everyone has learned to pronounce it.' (Bah-GO-tah, that is).[3]

●*AIDS.* Jill, a 26-year-old single woman from Wisconsin, says, 'AIDS has made casual sex out of the question. I take no chances. Sex is not worth dying for. I would only have sex now using a condom and with someone I'm seriously interested in. I would tell others simply that it's life or death. Take precautions or take the consequences.'[4]

●*AIDS.* Because of the threat of AIDS, the Los Angeles school district makes condoms available to students, with parental permission. Because of AIDS, the New York City school district hands out condoms to students without parental permission or parental knowledge.

●*AIDS.* Despite the availability of condoms in New York City schools, a 17-year-old male high-school student tells a reporter that he does not use one when he makes love to his 'girl.' When asked why, he explains, 'Because I love her too much.'[5]

●*AIDS.* Karen, a junior at an Ohio university, explains to an interviewer why she does not insist that her sex partners wear condoms when they make love: 'I have an attitude—it may be wrong—that any guy I would sleep with would not have AIDS.'[6]

●*AIDS.* During a protest march in Washington, D.C., in October 1987, the names of the first 1,000 AIDS victims are displayed on a quilt that stretches two blocks. The quilt eventually grows to be four miles long.

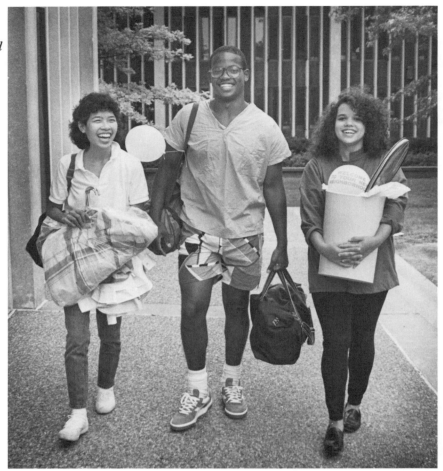

Coming of Age in the Age of AIDS. College is a time of exhilarating and sometimes stressful changes. Students sometimes jest that they are 'dying for sex,' but the advent of AIDS has meant that some people are literally dying because of their sexual behavior.

Coming of age can be a difficult thing. College is for many the opportunity of a lifetime—a ticket of admission to an education and a career. College can also be stressful, however. New students—especially those who attend college away from home—are removed from much that is familiar. They may face changes in eating and sleeping habits, the need to make new friends, and, often, more demanding academic work.

The college years bring new independence, and new independence means new responsibilities. It is during the college years that many students learn to manage their money and their time. Many

college students also have concerns left over from their high-school days. College students may worry about their physical stature—their athletic prowess and their body builds, and about their popularity with their peers. They may also wonder whether they are headed in the right direction, whether they are taking the right courses and aiming toward the proper career.

College students also tend to be concerned about sex and love. Social pressures at college may heighten conflict over sexual behavior. Many collegians remain concerned about some of the traditional questions: *Should* I? Now or later? Do

I have to be in love? What about pregnancy?

Two generations ago, after World War II, college students might also have been concerned about sexually transmitted diseases such as gonorrhea and syphilis. Syphilis is potentially life-threatening, but both gonorrhea and syphilis can be cured with antibiotics. A generation ago, during and shortly after the Vietnam War, students people were more likely to think about chlamydia and genital herpes. Chlamydia can go unnoticed, especially in women, until it results in infertility. Still, it is curable with antibiotics and not considered life-threatening. Genital herpes is painful and incurable, but it is not life-threatening to adults who contract the disease.

College students today still face the traditional sexual issues—the issues that touch on popularity, personal adequacy, and pregnancy.

College students still face gonorrhea, syphilis, chlamydia, and genital herpes.

For the first time, however, a generation of college students has come of age at a time when the threat of their own death hangs over every sexual encounter. Sex has become connected with a new concern—*AIDS*.

The notion of 'dying for sex' used to be an obvious overstatement. Today, however, people here and there are literally dying because they contracted AIDS through sexual activity.

Some students are more aware than others of the ways in which H.I.V. is transmitted and of the meaning of AIDS. The media brim with daily reports on H.I.V. and AIDS, but how much do you really know about them? The AIDS Awareness Inventory can help you find out.

The AIDS Awareness Inventory

To find out how much you know about H.I.V. and AIDS, place a T in the blank space for each item that you believe is true or mostly true. Place an F in the blank space for each item that you believe is false or mostly false. Then check your answers against the explanations offered in the pages that follow.

Before you get started, we want to issue a 'warning.' Some of the items in the questionnaire, and some of the content in the book, get at least an 'R' rating. If we were talking about a film, we would say that it contains some 'sex' and 'nudity.' There's no violence, however. The purpose of the questionnaire, like the purpose of this book, is to help you prevent doing violence to yourself.

___ 1. AIDS is synonymous with H.I.V. They are different names for the same thing.

___ 2. H.I.V. is a kind of bacteria.

___ 3. You can be infected with H.I.V. only by people who have AIDS.

___ 4. AIDS is a kind of pneumonia.

___ 5. AIDS is a form of cancer.

___ 6. You can't get infected with H.I.V. the first time you engage in sexual intercourse.

___ 7. You can't get AIDS if you are young and healthy.

___ 8. You can't get AIDS from someone who is young and healthy.

___ 9. You can't be infected by H.I.V. unless you're a homosexual or you inject ('shoot up') drugs.

___ 10. AIDS is more of a threat to men than to women.

___ 11. You can be infected by H.I.V. and not have any signs or symptoms of illness for many years.

12. You can be the most valuable player in the National Basketball Association All-Star Game and still be infected with H.I.V.

13. There are vaccines for AIDS.

14. You really don't have to worry about AIDS unless you live in places like New York or San Francisco, where there are lots of homosexuals and people who shoot up drugs.

15. You can't be infected with H.I.V. by hugging someone, even if that person is infected with H.I.V.

16. You can't be infected with H.I.V. by kissing someone, even if that person is infected with H.I.V.

17. You can't be infected with H.I.V. by having regular sexual intercourse (intercourse with the penis in the vagina), even if your partner is infected with H.I.V.

18. You can't be infected with H.I.V. through sexual activity if you're using contraception, even if your partner is infected with H.I.V.

19. You can't be infected with H.I.V. if you use a condom ('rubber,' 'safe') when you engage in sexual intercourse, even if your partner is infected with H.I.V.

20. You can't be infected with H.I.V. by oral sex (that is, from kissing, licking, or sucking a penis or a vagina), even if your partner is infected with H.I.V.

21. The World Health Organization estimates that 40 million people around the world are likely to be infected by H.I.V. by the year 2000.

22. The majority of people who have AIDS are homosexuals.

23. More than a million people in the United States have AIDS.

24. You can be infected with H.I.V. by donating blood.

25. If you already have a sexually transmitted disease, like chlamydia or genital warts, you can't be infected with H.I.V.

26. You can't be infected with H.I.V. if you and your sex partner are faithful to one another (don't have sex with anyone else).

27. Doctors and lab technicians determine whether or not people are infected with H.I.V. by examining their blood for H.I.V.

28. There are no medical treatments for H.I.V. infection or AIDS.

29. Knowledge of the risks of H.I.V. infection and AIDS causes people to abstain from sex or engage in 'safe sex.'

30. People are likely to be infected with H.I.V. if they are bitten by insects such as mosquitoes that are carrying it.

Now check your answers on the following pages.

Answers to the AIDS Awareness Inventory

How well did you do on the inventory? As you check the accuracy of your answers, you will come across a great deal of vocabulary that may be new to you—words and concepts ranging from *virus* to *injectable drug user* to *opportunistic infection*. These terms are all defined the first time they are used. They will be repeated throughout the book, and as you read, they will become more and more familiar.

When you are finished with the book you may not be a medical expert, but you will know the vocabulary you need to understand H.I.V.

infection and AIDS. Your knowledge may have greatly expanded, in fact, by the time you have read through the explanations for the answers to the inventory.

___ 1.   AIDS is synonymous with H.I.V. They are simply different names for the same thing.

False. AIDS is the name of a disease. AIDS stands for *acquired immune deficiency syndrome*. (A syndrome is a group of signs or symptoms of a disease.) H.I.V. stands for *human immunodeficiency virus*, which is the microscopic disease organism that causes AIDS. H.I.V. weakens the body's immune system—mainly the white blood cells that help you fight off diseases. When the immune system is weakened beyond a certain point, people are prey to illnesses that normally would not get a foothold in the body. At this time, they are said to have AIDS.

___ 2.   H.I.V. is a kind of bacteria.

False. H.I.V. is a kind of virus. Viruses are among the smallest microorganisms able to cause disease. Viruses can reproduce only within the cells of plants or animals.

___ 3.   You can be infected with H.I.V. only by people who have AIDS.

False. H.I.V. is transmitted by people who are infected with it, whether or not they have yet developed AIDS.

___ 4.   AIDS is a kind of pneumonia.

False. AIDS is a disease that is characterized by a weakened immune system. The name acquired immune deficiency syndrome means the immune system is deficient or inadequate. Because the immune system has been weakened, it no longer does its normal job of protecting us from disease. Because we are unprotected, we are apt to develop

illnesses that otherwise wouldn't stand much of a chance of taking hold. These illnesses are called 'opportunistic infections.' They take the opportunity to infect us, that is, because our immune systems are weakened. The confusion of AIDS with pneumonia may come about because one of these opportunistic illnesses happens to be a form of pneumonia, *Pneumocystis carinii pneumonia*—PCP for short. Before the emergence of AIDS, PCP was found only in cancer patients whose immune systems had been weakened, usually as a side effect of chemotherapy (therapy with chemicals or drugs). But AIDS itself is not a form of pneumonia.

___ 5.   AIDS is a form of cancer.

False. By now, you recognize that AIDS is a disease that is identified by a weakened immune system. Weakening of the immune system allows opportunistic illnesses to take hold. The confusion about AIDS and cancer may stem from the fact that men with weakened immune systems are prone to developing a rare form of skin cancer, *Kaposi's sarcoma*, which leaves purplish spots all over the body. Before the emergence of AIDS, this form of cancer had usually struck only aging Italian and Jewish men.

___ 6.   You can't get infected with H.I.V. the first time you engage in sexual intercourse.

False. Sure you can. There is a myth that you cannot become pregnant the first time you engage in sexual intercourse, but you most certainly can. Perhaps this erroneous belief about H.I.V. infection is connected with the myth about protection from pregnancy.

___ 7.   You can't get AIDS if you are young and healthy.

False. It would be nice to think that young, healthy people are immune to H.I.V. infection and AIDS!

Teenagers and young adults often consider themselves 'immune' to a variety of ills. Perhaps this is because many teenagers and young adults feel strong and healthy and see themselves as having countless years ahead of them. This sense of immunity encourages many teenagers to take foolish risks, however, such as driving recklessly. Reckless sex and drug use, unfortunately, can result in H.I.V. infection—regardless of how young and healthy one happens to be.

___ 8. You can't get AIDS from someone who is young and healthy.

False. By now, you probably realize that you do not 'get' AIDS from someone else; you are infected by H.I.V. and then you develop AIDS. More importantly, however, this statement is also false because you certainly can be infected by someone who is young and healthy. If that person is infected by H.I.V., she or he can infect you, even if she or he is on an Olympic team.

___ 9. You can't be infected by H.I.V. unless you're a homosexual or you inject ('shoot up') drugs.

False. You most certainly can be infected by H.I.V. without being a homosexual or shooting up drugs! It is true that homosexual men and people who inject drugs have been considered to be in high 'risk groups' for being infected by H.I.V., especially in the United States and Canada. (The risk in shooting up drugs comes from sharing needles with people who may be infected by H.I.V. The virus can contaminate the needle and then be spread to the bloodstreams of other users.) Everything else being equal, there is a greater chance that homosexual men and people who inject drugs (sometimes called 'injectable drug users' or 'IDU's') are infected by H.I.V. than most other groups are. But you become infected by H.I.V. by *doing* something, not by *being* something. *Anyone* can be infected by H.I.V. if the virus enters her or his bloodstream. For that reason, most health professionals are now talking about high-risk *behavior patterns* rather than high-risk *groups*.

___ 10. AIDS is more of a threat to men than to women.

False. As of today, more men than women have developed AIDS. This is largely because until now, H.I.V. was transmitted predominantly among homosexual males and people who injected drugs. The first group consists solely of males, and the second group is mostly male. The incidences of H.I.V. infection and AIDS are now growing more rapidly among women than men, however—in the United States and elsewhere. Women, moreover, are more vulnerable than men are to being infected with H.I.V. through sexual relations in which the penis is inserted in the vagina (heterosexual intercourse).

___ 11. You can be infected by H.I.V. and not have any signs or symptoms of illness for many years.

True. It is estimated that an average of about 10½ years passes between the time adolescents or adults are infected by H.I.V. and the time they develop AIDS.[7]

___ 12. You can be the most valuable player in the National Basketball Association All-Star Game and still be infected with H.I.V.

True. Absolutely true. Magic Johnson was the most valuable player of the all-star game in February 1992, three months after he retired from professional basketball because he learned that he had been infected by H.I.V. Does that mean that H.I.V. infection isn't anything to worry about? (After all, wouldn't we all like to be as strong and well-coordinated as the most valuable player in an all-star game?) Actually, medical authorities estimate that 99 percent of people infected with H.I.V. will eventually develop—and die

6

from—AIDS. From this point of view, Johnson has a time bomb in him that is waiting to go off. Don't be willing to trade places with Johnson or to expose yourself to H.I.V. because you believe that Johnson has a rosy future.

__ 13. There are vaccines for AIDS.

True and false—mostly false. A vaccine is given to confer immunity to a disease. You are vaccinated, that is, so that you will be protected from disease. It turns out that there are a number of *experimental* vaccines for H.I.V. and that at least one of them has been shown to give *monkeys* some protection against H.I.V. infection. No vaccine, however, has yet been shown to protect people from H.I.V. infection.

__ 14. You really don't have to worry about AIDS unless you live in places like New York or San Francisco, where there are lots of homosexuals and people who shoot up drugs.

False. You have to think about H.I.V. infection and AIDS regardless of where you live (and again, regardless of whether or not you have any connection with homosexual men or people who inject drugs). Remember that in 1992, 6 out of 197 students at rural Bogata, Texas's Rivercrest High School were reported to be infected with H.I.V. It is true that higher percentages of the population may be infected with H.I.V. in certain locations, but you can be infected with H.I.V. by just one person—and that person does not have to be a homosexual or a drug user.

__ 15. You can't be infected with H.I.V. by hugging someone, even if that person is infected with H.I.V.

True. In order to be infected with H.I.V., the virus must get into your bloodstream. This is unlikely to happen through hugging someone, even if that person is infected. This is why people who

care for H.I.V.-infected children can lavish affection on them without fear of being infected themselves.

__ 16. You can't be infected with H.I.V. by kissing someone, even if that person is infected with H.I.V.

False. Even though you may be right most of the time with this one, the statement is too general to be absolutely true. A peck on the cheek can be considered safe enough, but deep kissing (tongue kissing, soul kissing, French kissing) causes one person's saliva to enter the other person's mouth. H.I.V. has been found in the saliva of infected people. If there are little cuts in gums or elsewhere in the mouth—the sorts of minor cuts you may get from brushing your teeth or, perhaps, some kind of sores—it is conceivable that H.I.V. could enter your bloodstream in that way. There are a couple of reports that suggest that some people have been infected in this manner. Put it another way: we can't guarantee that tongue kissing with an infected person is safe, so you are advised to think about whom you kiss and, especially, *how* you kiss.

__ 17. You can't be infected with H.I.V. by having regular sexual intercourse (intercourse with the penis in the vagina), even if your partner is infected with H.I.V.

False. This erroneous belief may reflect the connection between homosexuality and AIDS in many people's minds. You most assuredly can be infected by H.I.V. in this manner, whether you are a woman or a man. Women are more likely than men to be infected in this way, in part because of the vulnerability of cells in the cervix to H.I.V. infection. Men can also be infected through vaginal intercourse, however, and many thousands have been, as we shall see—especially men who visit prostitutes. These men then often spread H.I.V. to their wives or girlfriends.

18. You can't be infected with H.I.V. through sexual activity if you're using contraception, even if your partner is infected with H.I.V.

False. You most certainly can. Some forms of contraception such as the birth-control pill and rhythm methods provide absolutely no protection against infection by H.I.V. Other methods such as spermicides provide some protection, but cannot be considered safe.

19. You can't be infected with H.I.V. if you use a condom ('rubber,' 'safe') when you engage in sexual intercourse, even if your partner is infected with H.I.V.

False. Condoms made of latex rubber do provide a good deal of protection against H.I.V. transmission. Condoms do not always work, however. Some condoms are torn or tear during use. Some people do not apply or remove them properly. Unfortunately, then, you *may* be infected by H.I.V. if you use a condom.

20. You can't be infected with H.I.V. by oral sex (that is, from kissing, licking, or sucking a penis or a vagina), even if your partner is infected with H.I.V.

False. It appears that you can be infected by H.I.V. through oral sex. This avenue of transmission is not very likely, in part because digestive juices (saliva and the normal acids that are found in the digestive tract) kill H.I.V. There appear to be a number of cases of people who have been infected in this manner, however.

21. The World Health Organization estimates that 40 million people around the world are likely to be infected by H.I.V. by the year 2000.

True. The WHO bases its projection on current patterns of transmission of H.I.V.

22. The majority of people who have AIDS are homosexuals.

False—with a qualifier. The statement is true within the United States and Canada, but not throughout the world. Even in the United States and Canada, homosexuals are accounting for fewer and fewer new cases of H.I.V. infection and AIDS. There is no doubt that people can be infected by H.I.V. by engaging in sexual intercourse with a member of the opposite sex. Within a few years, the majority of people who have been infected will probably have been infected through sexual intercourse with a member of the opposite sex.

23. More than a million people in the United States have AIDS.

False. It is estimated that more than a million people in the United States are infected with H.I.V., but only a fraction of this number have developed AIDS to date. Let us hope that we find a vaccine or cure before the great majority of these people—and others—do develop AIDS. If we don't, within a few years more than a million people in the United States will, in fact, have died of AIDS.

24. You can be infected with H.I.V. by donating blood.

False. It is not true that you can be infected by H.I.V. by donating blood. The needles are sterile (free of infection) and are used only once.

25. If you already have a sexually transmitted disease, like chlamydia or genital warts, you can't be infected with H.I.V.

False. Some people believe, erroneously, that they cannot be placed in 'double jeopardy' by sexually transmitted diseases. People who have another sexually transmitted disease are actually *more* likely, not less likely, to be infected by H.I.V. There are at least two reasons for this. One is that they may have sores in the genital region that provide convenient ports of entry for H.I.V. into the bloodstream. The second is that the risky sexual behavior that led to one kind of infection can easily lead to others.

___ 26. You can't be infected with H.I.V. if you and your sex partner are faithful to one another (don't have sex with anyone else).

False. You certainly cut your risks through a monogamous relationship, but you must consider two questions: The first is what your faithful partner was doing before the two of you became a couple. The second is whether or not your partner engages in some nonsexual form of behavior that could result in H.I.V. infection, such as shooting up drugs.

___ 27. Doctors and lab technicians determine whether or not people are infected with H.I.V. by examining their blood for H.I.V.

False. H.I.V. itself is difficult to detect, so H.I.V. infection is usually diagnosed by checking for *antibodies* to the virus in the bloodstream. Antibodies are chemicals that your own body manufactures when you have been invaded by a virus, bacteria, or other disease-causing agent. Antibodies fight off and protect your from most disease-causing organisms. This is not the case with H.I.V. unfortunately.

___ 28. There are no medical treatments for H.I.V. infection or AIDS.

False. There definitely are some medical treatments for H.I.V. and AIDS. There are drugs such as zidovudine that slow down the spread or multiplication of H.I.V. within the body, for example. There are also medications for many of

the 'opportunistic illnesses' that attack people who have developed AIDS. Other methods such as proper diet, rest, and stress management may also be of help. None of these methods eliminates H.I.V. infection from the body or cures AIDS, however. Although they may give at least temporary boosts to the immune system, questions also remain as to whether or not they actually prolong the lives of people who are infected with H.I.V. or who have developed AIDS.

Put it another way: Yes, there are medical (and other) treatments for H.I.V. infection and AIDS. It is not clear how effective they are, however.

___ 29. Knowledge of the risks of H.I.V. infection and AIDS causes people to abstain from sex or engage in 'safe sex.'

False. Would that it were so! Unfortunately, many if not most people who are educated about H.I.V. and AIDS still engage in behavior that places them at risk of infection.

___ 30. People are likely to be infected with H.I.V. if they are bitten by insects such as mosquitoes that are carrying it.

False! Apparently you do not have to be concerned about the insects that mill about in next summer's heated air. Even though it is theoretically possible that an insect that drinks the blood of several people could transmit H.I.V., there is no documented case of H.I.V. having been transmitted in this manner.

If you answered each of the questions correctly, you can stop reading right here. In fact, you—and not we—should have written this book. If you answered some of the items incorrectly, we advise reading on—for your own sake and for the sake of the people you care about.

2 AIDS
—The First Decade

Many of you may remember where you were and what you were doing on November 7, 1991. That's the day that Los Angeles Laker Magic Johnson, who had led his team to five NBA championships, retired from professional basketball. He retired because he learned that he had been infected by the *human immunodeficiency virus* (H.I.V.). H.I.V. is the virus that causes *acquired immune deficiency syndrome* (AIDS).

Johnson said that he had been infected through heterosexual intercourse (sexual relations with a person of the opposite sex). He did not know when and with whom, however. Magic had not yet developed AIDS, and he is being treated with antiviral drugs that might slow the reproduction of H.I.V. Although he was free of symptoms at the time, his prospects looked grim. Researchers believe that perhaps 99 percent of people infected with the virus will eventually develop AIDS.

Magic Johnson's disclosure of his H.I.V. status may well have more impact in raising public awareness about H.I.V. and AIDS than the death of actor Rock Hudson from AIDS a few years earlier, especially among young people and minority youth in particular. Johnson's infection contributed to the shattering of the myth that young, strong boys and men who engage in sexual relations with women are invulnerable to H.I.V. If H.I.V. could strike Magic Johnson, it could strike anyone. Johnson's announcement had an immediate impact in raising awareness, and concerns, about H.I.V. and AIDS.

In the month following Johnson's announcement, the number of people requesting H.I.V. tests increased sharply across the country. Some cities reported a tenfold increase. The Centers for Disease Control in Atlanta reported that the number of calls to its toll-free AID hotline (800-342-2437) increased to 25,000 a day, compared to 3,000 to 5,000 before the nation learned of Johnson's infection.

Johnson's press conference is one of the landmarks in the brief history of AIDS. If Johnson had been infected only ten years earlier, no one would have thought to test for it. In fact, there would have been no test to reveal the infection. Moreover, the disease caused by that infection would not yet have had a name. The 'time line' on the following pages chronicles some of the major events of the first decade during which AIDS was recognized. Note that because of the high early incidence of the disease among homosexual ('gay') men, it was first called GRID, for gay-related immune deficiency.

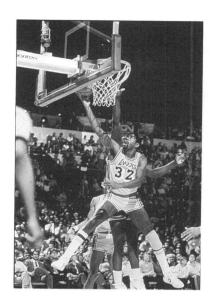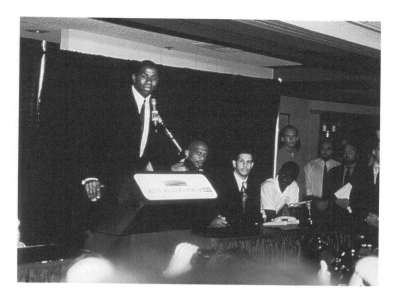

Magic Johnson on the Court and at His Press Conference on November 7, 1991. During his dozen years on the court, Los Angeles Laker Magic Johnson had led his team to five championships. On November 7, 1991, he announced his retirement from professional basketball because he learned that he had been infected by human immunodeficiency virus (HIV), the virus that causes acquired immune deficiency syndrome (AIDS). Prior to Johnson's announcement, many Americans had believed that only homosexuals and people who injected ('shot up') drugs were at serious risk of infection. Johnson's courageous public admission highlighted the fact that heterosexual, non-drug-abusing people are also at risk. One's behavior, and not one's group membership, places one at risk of HIV infection and AIDS.

AIDS—THE FIRST DECADE: A TIME LINE

1981

Ronald Reagan is inaugurated as the 40th president of the United States. Fifty-two hostages being held at the U.S. Embassy in Tehran, Iran, are released.

Washington defeats the Miami Dolphins in the Super Bowl, 21–17.
The Boston Celtics win the National Basketball Association championship.
The L.A. Dodgers defeat the New York Yankees in the World Series, 4 games to 2.

John Hinckley shoots President Reagan in an assassination attempt.

The first U.S. space shuttle, Columbia, makes a successful maiden flight.

The 'PC' is born. IBM Corporation launches its 'personal computer'—also known as the 'home computer.'

Israel destroys an Iraqi nuclear plant in an air attack near Baghdad, and the U.N. Security Council unanimously condemns the attack. (In the fall of 1990, after Saddam Hussein's Iraq invaded Kuwait, more than 60 percent of Americans said that they would be willing to go to war with Iraq to prevent Hussein from obtaining nuclear weapons.)

Anwar Sadat, the president of Egypt, is assassinated.

Muhammad Ali retires from professional boxing.

The Oscar for the best picture of 1980 is given to *Ordinary People*.

John Lennon and Yoko Ono win a Grammy award for the best album, *Double Fantasy*.

In June, the Federal Centers for Disease Control (CDC) reports a rare form of pneumonia (Pneumocystis carinii pneumonia, or PCP) in five homosexual (gay) men.

One month later, the CDC reports more mysterious illnesses in gay men.

The CDC reports 152 cases of what it is now calling GRID (gay-related immune deficiency).

1982

The Los Angeles Raiders defeat Washington, 38–9, in the Super Bowl.

St. Louis Cardinals defeat the Milwaukee Brewers in the World Series, 4 games to 3.

The Boston Celtics repeat as the NBA champions.

Leonid Brezhnev, the leader of the Soviet Union dies and is succeeded by KGB chief Yuri Andropov.

Helmut Kohl becomes chancellor of West Germany.

Israel returns the Sinai peninsula to Egypt, in accord with the Camp David peace treaty.

EPCOT Center (the acronym for 'Experimental Community of Tomorrow') opens at Disney World in Florida.

The Oscar for the best picture of 1981 is given to *Chariots of Fire*.

Popular songs of 1981 include *Rosanna*, *Truly*, and *Up Where We Belong*.

A CDC publication suggests that GRID is an infectious disease that is spread among sexual partners.

Over the summer, the CDC reports cases of the new disease in hemophiliacs and Haitian immigrants. The name GRID is changed to AIDS (acquired immune deficiency syndrome).

At year's end, the CDC reports 1,300 cases of AIDS in the United States and 317 deaths caused by AIDS (see Figure 2.1).

1983

Washington defeats the Miami Dolphins, 21–17, in the Super Bowl.

The Baltimore Orioles defeat the Philadelphia Phillies in the World Series, 4 games to 1.

The Philadelphia 76ers win the NBA championship.

President Reagan signs legislation to make Martin Luther King, Jr.'s birthday a national holiday from January 1986 onward.

Barney Clark, the first patient to receive an artificial heart, dies twelve days later.

The TV series *M*A*S*H* comes to an end.

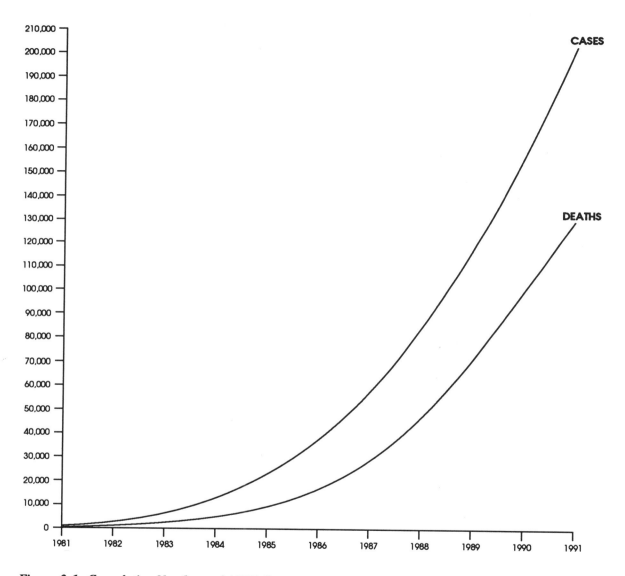

Figure 2.1. Cumulative Numbers of AIDS Cases and Deaths Caused by AIDS in the United States at the End of Each Year During the First Decade of the Epidemic, as Reported by the Centers for Disease Control.

Sally Ride is the first U.S. woman in space;
  Guion Bluford is the first African-
  American astronaut.
The Oscar for the best picture of 1982 is given
  to *Gandhi*. The film *Flashdance*
  popularizes the wiry, muscular look in
  women.
Popular songs of the year include *Beat It*,
  Thriller, *Flashdance*, and *Every Breath
  You Take*.

*The first cases of AIDS among heterosexuals
are reported by the CDC.*

*In March, people at high risk of being
infected with H.I.V. are asked not to donate
blood.*

*One month later, the first AIDS cover story
appears in* Newsweek.

*In the late spring, AIDS is declared the
'Number 1 health priority' in the nation.*

*During the summer, a French team headed
by Dr. Luc Montagnier finds a previously
unknown virus in AIDS patients.*

*At year's end, the CDC reports 4,156 cases
of AIDS in the United States. There are now
1,291 deaths.*

1984

The Los Angeles Raiders defeat Washington,
  38–9, in the Super Bowl.
The Detroit Tigers defeat the San Diego Padres
  in the World Series, 4 games to 1.
The Boston Celtics are the NBA champions.
Ronald Reagan is elected to his second term as
  president.
The PG–13 rating is created by the Motion
  Picture Association of America for films
  that are too mild for the R rating but a
  bit too saucy for PG.
The Disney empire celebrates the 50th birthday
  of Donald Duck.

The Oscar for the best picture of 1983 is given
  to the Debra Winger tearjerker, *Terms
  of Endearment*. Other popular films that
  come out in 1984 include *Ghostbusters*
  and *Beverly Hills Cop*—the originals,
  not the sequels.
Michael Jackson wins an unprecedented eight
  Grammy awards for his *Thriller* album,
  which also sells 38 million copies.

*In April, H.I.V., the virus that causes AIDS,
is clearly identified by a U.S. research team
headed by Dr. Robert Gallo of the National
Cancer Institute.*

*At year's end, the CDC reports 9,920 cases
of AIDS in the United States and 3,665 deaths
to date.*

1985

The San Francisco 49ers defeat the Miami
  Dolphins, 38–16, in the Super Bowl.
The Kansas City Royals defeat the St. Louis
  Cardinals, 4 games to 1, in the World
  Series.
The Los Angeles Lakers win the NBA
  championship.
Pete Rose of the Cincinnati Reds gets his 4,192th
  career hit, tying Ty Cobb's record.
Mikhail Gorbachev becomes the general
  secretary of the Soviet Union's
  Communist Party.
The Oscar for the best picture of 1984 is given
  to *Amadeus*.
The song *We Are the World*, written by Lionel
  Richie and Michael Jackson, is sung by
  a group including Cindy Lauper and
  Bruce Springsteen, to benefit hungry
  Ethiopian children.

Early in the year, Luc Montagnier (the head of the French research team) and Robert Gallo (the Head of the U.S. research team) decide to share the credit for discovering the AIDS virus—H.I.V. (human immunodeficiency virus).

In March, a test for H.I.V. antibodies is licensed by the Federal Drug Administration.

The first international AIDS conference is held in Atlanta, Georgia.

In the early fall, a poll finds that one out of four people in the United States believe that children with AIDS should not be allowed in schools.

At year's end, a cumulative total of 20,470 U.S. AIDS cases is reported by the CDC. There are 8,161 deaths to date.

1986

The Chicago Bears defeat the New England Patriots, 46–10, in the Super Bowl. Bears defensive lineman 'Refrigerator' Perry captures the public imagination as a running back on short-yardage touchdown plays.

The New York Mets defeat the Boston Red Sox, 4 games to 3, in the World Series.

The Boston Celtics are the NBA champions.

The space shuttle Challenger explodes during lift-off. All seven passengers, including New Hampshire schoolteacher Christa McAuliffe, die.

Mike Tyson becomes the WBC world heavyweight boxing champion. In 1992, Tyson would be convicted of the date rape of an 18-year-old beauty pageant contestant.

The Oscar for the best picture of 1985 is given to *Out of Africa*, which stars Meryl Streep and Robert Redford.

The Broadway musical *Les Miserables* wins eight Tony awards.

Whitney Houston and Madonna sit atop the popular music charts.

Early in the year, researchers announce that the AIDS virus can lie dormant for years.

In the summer, the second international AIDS conference is held.

In the fall Surgeon General Dr. C. Everett Koop calls for explicit education about H.I.V. infection and AIDS and for use of condoms.

At year's end, the CDC reports a cumulative total of 37,061 U.S. AIDS cases; there are 16,301 deaths to date.

1987

The New York Giants defeat the Denver Broncos, 39–20, in the Super Bowl. Giants quarterback Phil Simms completes 22 of 25 passes.

The Minnesota Twins defeat the St. Louis Cardinals, 4 games to 3, in the World Series.

The Los Angeles Lakers win the NBA championship.

The issue of surrogate motherhood explodes on the national scene with the Baby M trial, in which Mary Beth Whitehead loses custody of her child.

On October 19th, 'Black Monday,' the final leg of the 'Crash of 87' occurs as the Dow Jones Industrial Average of the New York Stock Exchange plummets 508 points. Some 1,000 points have been lost since the new top of 2,722 points was reached in August 1987.

Mikhail Gorbachev campaigns in the Soviet Union for *glasnost* (openness) and *perestroika* (economic restructuring).

Former Senator Gary Hart withdraws from the race for the Democratic nomination for the presidency after reports of an affair with model Donna Rice. Photos of Rice in Hart's lap aboard the boat Monkey Business are made public, and Rice goes on to model No Excuses blue jeans in an advertising campaign.

The Oscar for the best picture of 1986 is given to *Platoon*.
Popular songs include *Graceland*, *Bad*, and *Higher Love*.

In the spring, the AIDS Coalition to Unleash Power (ACT-UP) is formed in New York City by AIDS activists. Their slogan is Silence = Death.

In the same month, AZT (which is now called zidovudine) is the first AIDS drug to approved by the FDA.

The third international AIDS conference is held.

During an autumn protest march in Washington, DC, the names of the first 1,000 AIDS victims are displayed on a quilt that stretches two blocks. The quilt eventually grows to be four miles long.

At year's end, 59,587 U.S. AIDS cases are reported; there are 27,909 deaths to date.

1988

Washington defeats the Denver Broncos in the Super Bowl, 42–10.
The Los Angeles Dodgers defeat the Oakland Athletics in the World Series, 4 games to 1. Dodgers pitcher Orel Hersheiser emerges as the series hero.
The Detroit Pistons are the NBA champions.
George Bush is elected to the 41st president.
Mikhail Gorbachev becomes president of the Soviet Union.
The Oscar for the best picture of 1987 is given to *The Last Emperor*.
Popular films of the year include *Big*, *Die Hard*, *The Naked Gun*, and *Rain Man*.
Popular songs include *Don't Worry, Be Happy*, *Faith*, and *Fast Car*.

During the summer, the fourth international AIDS conference is held in Stockholm, Sweden.
At year's end, there are 88,864 cases of AIDS reported in the United States; there are 46,134 deaths to date.

1989

The San Francisco 49ers defeat the Cincinnati Bengals, 20–16, in the Super Bowl.
The Oakland Athletics defeat the San Francisco Giants, 4 games to none, in a World Series that is punctuated by the San Francisco Earthquake of 1989, which kills sixty-seven people and does extensive damage to the Bay Area.
The Detroit Pistons win the NBA championship.
The Berlin Wall is torn down, ushering in free movement in Berlin and between East and West Germany. (The Soviet Union announces that it no longer interferes in the internal affairs of other nations.)
Candidates from Poland's noncommunist Solidarity movement win an overwhelming majority of seats in parliament.
General Manuel Noriega, the ruler of Panama, annuls the results of a free election that is won by an opposition candidate. The United States invades Panama, brings Noriega to the United States to stand trial for smuggling drugs into the United States, and installs a new government in Panama.
Eleven million gallons of oil are spilled onto the coastline of Alaska when the Exxon Valdez oil tanker runs aground.
Hurricane Hugo does extensive damage in the Caribbean and to the coastline of South Carolina.
The Oscar for best picture of 1988 is won by *Rain Man*.
Popular films of 1989 include *Batman* and *Look Who's Talking*.

16

The top record albums of the year include *Don't be Cruel* (Bobby Brown), *Hangin' Tough* (New Kids on the Block), *Forever Your Girl* (Paula Abdul), and *New Jersey* (Bon Jovi).

In February, the Federal Drug Administration (FDA) grants limited approval of aerosol pentamidine to prevent PCP, which kills about 60 percent of AIDS patients.

During the summer, the fifth international AIDS conference is held in Montreal, Canada.

Also during the summer, researchers report studies that show that AZT slows, but does not stop, H.I.V. progression. Some people cry out for mandatory testing for the AIDS virus, but AIDS activists endorse voluntary testing only.

At year's end, the CDC reports a total of 115,756 U.S. AIDS cases to date; the cumulative total of AIDS-related deaths now stands at 70,313.

1990

The San Francisco 49ers defeat the Denver Broncos, 55–10, in the Super Bowl. Having won two consecutive Super Bowls, team members adopt the slogan that they will 'three-peat' next year. Joe Montana is hailed as the best quarterback who ever played the game, and the Montana–Jerry Rice passing combination is considered unstoppable.

The underdog Cincinnati Reds defeat the Oakland Athletics, 4 games to none, in the World Series.

The Detroit Pistons win the NBA championship.

Germany is officially reunified. Helmut Kohl presides as the first chancellor of the united Germany.

Iraq occupies Kuwait on August 2.

Mikhail Gorbachev wins the Nobel Peace Prize as Soviet hard-liners want to know, 'Who lost Eastern Europe?'

The Oscar for best picture of 1989 is won by *Driving Miss Daisy*. Whoopi Goldberg wins the award for best supporting actress in the film *Ghost*.

The Madonna video *Justify My Love* is barred from being shown on MTV.

During the summer, the sixth international AIDS conference is held. AIDS activists and scientists try to develop a mutually satisfactory system for getting promising new treatments to AIDS patients, even before they gain approval through normal channels at the FDA.

At year's end, the CDC reports a total of 161,073 U.S. AIDS cases; there are 100,813 deaths to date.

1991

The New York Giants defeat the Buffalo Bills in the Super Bowl, 20–19, when Buffalo misses a field goal in the waning seconds of the game. Back-up quarterback Jeff Hosteteler performs late-season heroics in the stead of the Giants' injured Phil Simms.

The Minnesota Twins defeat Atlanta, 4 games to 3, in the World Series. Native Americans protest that the Atlanta team name ('Braves') and the fans' 'tomahawk chop' degrades them.

The Chicago Bulls ride to the NBA championship via 'Air Jordan'—Michael Jordan, that is.

On January 16, the United States and allied nations attack Iraq, initiating the 'War in the Gulf.' Generals 'Stormin' Norman' Schwarzkopf and Colin Powell capture the public imagination. After his defeat, allied forces allow Saddam Hussein to remain in power in Iraq. In the wake of the stunning U.S.-led victory, President George Bush's approval rating soars to about 90 percent.

The Oscar for best picture of 1990 is given to *Dances with Wolves.*

The Grammy award for record of the year goes to *Another Day in Paradise* (Phil Collins). The award for song of the year is given to *From a Distance*, which is sung by Bette Midler.

Mikhail Gorbachev is placed under house arrest in the Crimea in an August coup by Communist hard-liners. The coup fails largely because of the heroics of Russian President Boris Yeltsin, and Gorbachev is returned to his position as president of the Soviet Union.

As a recession continues in the United States, George Bush's approval rating plummets to about 47 percent by year's end.

On December 31, despite the efforts of Gorbachev to hold the Soviet Union together, the nations that comprise the union—largely at the urging of Yeltsin—decide to go their separate ways. Gorbachev is out of a job. (In February 1992, Gorbachev's first editorial column would appear in *The New York Times.*)

June is the tenth anniversary of the first AIDS report by the CDC. The seventh international AIDS conference is held. At the conference, it is estimated 1 million people in the United States are infected with H.I.V. The World Health Organization (WHO) estimates that 10 million people are infected worldwide and projects that 40 million will be infected by the year 2000.

A second drug, dideoxyinosine (DDI), is approved for use in treating AIDS, even though it is still in the experimental stage of development and requires further testing.

On November 7, Magic Johnson announces his retirement from professional basketball because he is infected with H.I.V. Johnson says that he was infected through heterosexual sex and urges young people to practice safe sex. In response to criticism for urging safe sex, Johnson suggests sexual abstinence and monogamy as alternatives for young people a few weeks later.

At year's end, more than 202,000 U.S. AIDS cases are reported by the CDC; there are more than 130,000 deaths to date (see Figure 2.1). ■

The remainder of this chapter recounts some of the events in the brief history of AIDS more closely.

In 1981, Michael Gottlieb, a young physician at the University of California at Los Angeles, treated several patients who were suffering from a rare form of pneumonia, *Pneumocystis carinii pneumonia* (PCP). PCP had previously been found only among cancer patients who showed suppressed immune systems, usually as a result of *chemotherapy.* Several other men appeared at UCLA, also suffering from PCP as well as from mysterious high fevers, weight loss, and other unusual features associated with a depleted immunological system, such as *candidiasis* (a yeast infection) of the mouth. Gottlieb expected that the men would recover. But he was wrong. They all died.

Gottlieb was the first physician to report this unusual array of symptoms in the medical literature. At the time, it was a syndrome without a name. Within a few years, however, it would come to be called AIDS. Researchers would later discover that the earliest known case of AIDS in the United States occurred in a teenage boy in St. Louis in 1968. Although the origins of H.I.V. remain unclear, it is widely believed that related strains of the virus probably originated in monkeys and chimpanzees in Africa. Scientists have found a similar virus in a West African monkey. In an intriguing but unproven hypothesis, some scientists suspect that the virus was introduced in humans as the unintended result of malaria experiments dating from the 1920s to the 1950s. In those experiments, people were inoculated with blood from monkeys and chimpanzees that may have contained viral ancestors of H.I.V. The purpose of the experiments was to see whether malaria parasites in these animals would infect humans.

In 1981, fewer than 100 people in the United States had died of AIDS. By the end of 1991, AIDS would be reported in more than 202,000 people in the United States and cause more than 130,000 U.S. deaths. By 1989, AIDS and H.I.V.-related infections had become the second leading cause of death in the United States among men aged 25 to 44, accounting for 14 percent of deaths among men in this group. By 1990, one death from AIDS occurred every 12 minutes in the United States. In 1990, at least 1 million Americans and 10 million people worldwide were infected with H.I.V. By the year 2000, the World Health Organization estimates that some 40 million people worldwide will be infected with H.I.V. Ten million will have developed AIDS. Figure 2.2 shows the estimated global distribution of adult H.I.V. infections in 1991. As you can see, Africa has been hardest hit to date.

Each year, 1,500 to 2,000 babies born in the United States are believed to be infected with H.I.V. AIDS has become the leading cause of death of Hispanic-American children 1 to 4 years of age, and the second leading killer of African-American children in that age range in New York City.

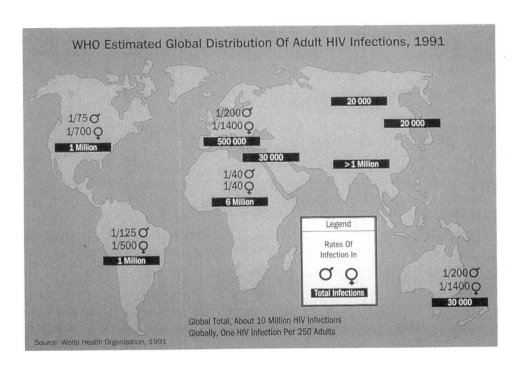

Figure 2.2. The World Health Organization's Estimate of the Global Distribution of Adult H.I.V. Infections in 1991. Africa has been hardest hit to date.

Some communities, especially inner-city neighborhoods with large numbers of people who inject ('shoot up') drugs, have been especially hard hit. In New York City, for example, as many as 60 percent of the people who are estimated to inject drugs (IDUs) are believed to be infected with H.I.V.

Researchers fear that the worst is yet to come. The numbers of AIDS cases and the resulting death toll are expected to increase through at least the 1990s. By the time this book is published, public health officials expect that AIDS will be diagnosed in 390,000 to 480,000 people in the United States and will have claimed 285,000 to 340,000 lives (see Table 2.1).

Physicians in the early 1980s also began seeing cases of young men with a rare cancer of the blood cells, *Kaposi's sarcoma*. Some also had PCP (*Pneumocystis carinii pneumonia*).

These men and those examined by Gottlieb had one thing in common: they were all gay. The syndrome without a name was soon dubbed the 'gay plague' or the 'gay cancer.' Social critics contend that the government initially responded slowly to the epidemic because of prejudice against homosexuals. According to journalist Randy Shilts[1], the nation did not take full notice of AIDS until high-profile celebrities—movie star Rock Hudson, fashion designer Perry Ellis, and choreographer Michael Bennett, among scores of others—contracted and died of AIDS:

> By October 2, 1985, the morning Rock Hudson died, the word was familiar to almost every household in the Western world.
> AIDS.
> Acquired Immune Deficiency Syndrome had seemed a comfortably distant threat to most of these who had heard of it before, the misfortune of people who fit into rather distinct classes of outcasts and social pariahs.

But suddenly, in the summer of 1985, when a movie star was diagnosed with the disease and the newspapers couldn't stop talking about it, the AIDS epidemic became palpable and the threat loomed everywhere.

Suddenly there were children with AIDS who wanted to go to school, laborers with AIDS who wanted to work, and researchers who wanted funding, and there was a threat to the nation's public health that could not longer be ignored. Most significantly, there were the first glimmers of awareness that the future would always contain this strange new word. AIDS would become a part of [U.S.] culture and indelibly change the course of our lives. . . .

Rock Hudson riveted [the attention of the United States] upon this deadly new threat . . . , and his diagnosis became a demarcation that would separate the history of [the United States] before AIDS from the history that came after.

The 'gay plague' began to strike heterosexuals, mostly people who inject drugs, their sex partners, babies born to infected mothers, and hemophiliacs (who had received transfusions of contaminated blood). AIDS was no longer a condition that afflicted only homosexuals. It became evident that the virus that causes AIDS did not know or care that the body it invaded belonged to a homosexual, heterosexual, or a newborn baby.

The best-known AIDS activist group, the AIDS Coalition to Unleash Power (ACT-UP) was founded in 1987 and further focused attention on the epidemic. ACT-UP's tactics can be highly abrasive, and some members of the medical establishment were turned off by them. According to Dr. Robert M. Wachter[2] of the University of California at San Francisco Medical School:

Table 2.1
Actual and Projected Number of AIDS Cases in the United States

YEAR	NEW CASES[a]	NUMBER LIVING[b]	DEATHS
1989	44,000–50,000	92,000–98,000	31,000–34,000
1990	52,000–57,000	101,000–122,000	37,000–42,000
1991	56,000–71,000	127,000–153,000	43,000–52,000
1992	58,000–85,000	139,000–188,000	49,000–64,000
1993	61,000–98,000	151,000–225,000	53,000–76,000
Through 1993	390,000–480,000		285,000–340,000

[a]Number of cases diagnosed during the year.
[b]Persons with AIDS alive during the year.
Source of data: Centers for Disease Control. (1990). Progress toward achieving the 1990 objectives for the nation for sexually transmitted diseases. *Morbidity and Mortality Weekly Report, 39,* 53–57.

[The] entry of AIDS activists into the health care scene has added a jarring new dimension to what was previously a genteel dialogue between patient advocates and clinicians, researchers, and policy makers. The activists' unprecedented modus operandi is a study in contrasts: street theater and intimidation on the one hand, detailed position papers and painstaking negotiation on the other. The effect has been to energize the fight against AIDS with an urgency that has translated into expedited [government] drug approvals, lower prices for medications, and increased funding for AIDS research and care.

AIDS activists maintain, of course, that when one is faced with death, the loss of a 'genteel dialogue' is no loss at all. They argue that the energizing of the battle against AIDS is basic to the survival of millions of people worldwide. In the early years of the final decade of the twentieth century, AIDS activists and a government commission (the National Commission on AIDS) *agreed* that the government had still not provided the funding support needed for AIDS research, prevention, and treatment. Michael Gottlieb[3] noted that:

> I don't think we have done all that we could be doing to prevent the spread of this virus, particularly in minority populations. What was a limited outbreak in the early 1980s has become

the holocaust we are facing because of politically motivated hang-ups [that have reduced the government's efforts] to prevent transmission.

Without a magic bullet and with the current low levels of prevention efforts, this [H.I.V.] virus will remain endemic well into the next century. This has happened in a first-world country in an era of unprecedented technology that could have been used by the public health sector to prevent such a disaster. That represents a failure that we should learn a lesson from.

Will the epidemic still be upon us as we enter the third millennium A.D.? Have we thus far seen only the tip of the iceberg, or will we make strides in the prevention and treatment of H.I.V. infection and AIDS?

3 AIDS and the Immune System

You might think that you depend on doctors and other highly trained specialists to cope with invading disease organisms and illnesses. At times you do, of course, but most of the time you defeat disease organisms by yourself, through a natural line of body defenses, part of which is your *immune system*.

AIDS is caused by the *human immunodeficiency virus* (H.I.V.)—a virus that strikes the body's immune system. Let us describe the ways in which your body protects you from diseases in general, so that you will better understand the kind of damage that is done by H.I.V.

WAYS IN WHICH THE BODY DEFENDS ITSELF AGAINST DISEASE

Numerous parts of your body protect you from disease. These include your skin, your mouth, your respiratory tract, your urinary tract, your gastrointestinal tract, and your bloodstream (see Table 3.1).

H.I.V. must get into the bloodstream to do its damage. The skin normally serves as a barrier to H.I.V. and other disease-causing organisms. If infected saliva, blood, vaginal fluid, or *semen* (semen is the thick, whitish fluid that is produced by the male reproductive organs and that carries sperm) is on your skin, H.I.V. will usually die there or remain there until it is washed away. A cut on the skin could allow H.I.V. into your bloodstream, however.

If infected saliva, blood, vaginal fluid, or semen gets into your mouth, some of it will be washed away. But if there are small cuts in your mouth from cold sores or brushing your teeth, H.I.V. could get into your bloodstream. If swallowed, most of the H.I.V. in infected saliva, blood, vaginal fluid, and semen will be destroyed by the acid in the gastrointestinal tract.

Let us now see what happens when H.I.V. gets into the bloodstream. To do so, we must explain how the immune system works.

Table 3.1
WAYS IN WHICH THE BODY DEFENDS ITSELF AGAINST DISEASE

Area of Defense from Disease-Causing Organisms	Defense Mechanisms in the Area	How the Defense Mechanisms Work	Factors That Can Weaken the Defenses
Skin	Intact skin surface	Provides a mechanical barrier to microorganisms	Cuts, abrasions, puncture wounds
	Shedding of outer layer of skin cells	Removes microorganisms that cling to the skin's outer layer	Failure to wash regularly
Mouth	Intact mucus lining	Provides a mechanical barrier to microorganisms	Cuts, extracted teeth
	Saliva	Washes away particles containing microorganisms	Poor oral hygiene, dryness
Respiratory tract	Hairlike projections from cells (cilia) that line the airways, which have a sticky mucus coating	Cilia trap microorganisms that are breathed in and sweep them out in mucus to be spit out or swallowed	Smoking, elevated concentrations of oxygen and carbon dioxide, cold dry air
	Cells (called macrophages) that ingest and destroy foreign agents	Engulf and destroy microorganisms that reach the lungs	Smoking
Urinary tract	Urine flow	Flushes away microorganisms in the urethra or the bladder	Obstruction in the urinary tract; delayed urination
	Intact lining of the tract	Provides barrier to microorganisms	Foreign objects in the urinary tract
Gastrointestinal tract	Acidity of gastric secretions	Chemically destroys many disease-causing microorganisms	Antacids (Tums, Rolaids, and so forth)
	Rapid rhythmic, wavelike movements (called peristalsis) of the walls of the intestines	Sweeps microorganisms out of body in bowel movements	Constipation, obstructions
Circulatory system	Cells (called macrophages) that ingest and destroy foreign agents	Engulf and destroy microorganisms that reach the bloodstream	Steroids, stress, *human immunodeficiency virus (H.I.V.)*

AIDS AND THE IMMUNE SYSTEM

THE IMMUNE SYSTEM

Your immune system combats disease in many ways. It produces white blood cells that engulf and destroy disease-causing organisms such as bacteria, viruses, and fungi. Disease-causing organisms are called *pathogens*. The white blood cells also engulf and devour worn out body cells and cells that have become cancerous. White blood cells are called *lymphocytes*. Lymphocytes are the primary strike force of the immune system. They go on search-and-destroy missions in your bloodstream. Some lymphocytes mark pathogens for destruction. Other lymphocytes destroy them (see Figure 3.1).

Pathogens have different shapes, and lymphocytes recognize them according to the contours of their surfaces. The surfaces of disease-causing organisms (pathogens) are called *antigens*. Antigen is short for *anti*body *gen*erator. The immune system reacts to antigens by forming special proteins, or *antibodies*.

(The antigens are parts of the invading organisms. The antibodies are produced by you as a response to the antigens.) The antibodies attach to the invading organisms and mark them for destruction by other lymphocytes. (Infection by H.I.V. is usually diagnosed by examining the blood for the presence of H.I.V. *antibodies*—not H.I.V. itself.)

Some white blood cells are called 'memory cells.' Memory cells can remain in the bloodstream for many years. Memory cells form the basis for a quick immune response to an invader the second time around. The formation of memory cells is the reason that we can develop *permanent immunity* to many disease-causing organisms. Even though people can become very ill from the organisms that cause mumps, smallpox, and measles the first time they are infected, survivors may never fall prey to them again.

HUMAN IMMUNODEFICIENCY VIRUS (H.I.V.) AND THE IMMUNE SYSTEM

Viruses are among the smallest organisms that can cause disease in living things. They consist of a bit of genetic material in a protein coating. Viruses are also among the most primitive forms of life. They are so primitive that some scientists argue that they are not alive at all. Alive or not, they can threaten the lives of animals and plants that are trillions of times their size.

Although viruses are powerful enough to do a great deal of harm, they cannot reproduce on their own. They can only reproduce (or 'multiply') within the cells of their living plant or animal hosts—including human hosts. When viruses invade a cell in the body, they can direct the cell's

own reproductive machinery to spin off new viral particles, which then spread to other cells. The virus provides the genetic code that is needed for replication, and the host cell provides the necessary energy and raw materials for new viral particles. There are more than 200 known viruses that can cause disease in people. Some of these diseases are mild, and the host will almost always recover completely from the illness. Other diseases caused by viruses are some of the most dangerous diseases known.

One attack of viral diseases such as mumps, smallpox, and measles gives a person permanent immunity. With many diseases caused by viruses,

CELL WARS

About one trillion strong, our white blood cells constitute a highly specialized army of defenders, the most important of which are depicted here in a typical battle against a formidable enemy.

VIRUS
Needing help to spring to life, a virus is little more than a package of genetic information that must commandeer the machinery of a host cell to permit its own replication.

MACROPHAGE
Housekeeper and frontline defender, this cell engulfs and digests debris that washes into the bloodstream. Encountering a foreign organism, it summons helper T cells to the scene.

HELPER T CELL
As a commander in chief of the immune system, it identifies the enemy and rushes to the spleen and lymph nodes, where it stimulates the production of other cells to fight the infection.

KILLER T CELL
Recruited and activated by helper T cells, it specializes in killing cells of the body that have been invaded by foreign organisms as well as cells that have turned cancerous.

B CELL
Biologic arms factory, it resides in the spleen or the lymph nodes, where it is induced to replicate by helper T cells and then to produce potent chemical weapons called antibodies.

ANTIBODY
Engineered to target a specific invader, this Y-shaped protein molecule is rushed to the infection site, where it either neutralizes the enemy or tags it for attack by other cells or chemicals.

SUPPRESSOR T CELL
A third type of T cell, it is able to slow down or stop the activities of B cells and other T cells, playing a vital role in calling off the attack after an infection has been conquered.

MEMORY CELL
Generated during an initial infection, this defense cell may circulate in the blood or lymph for years, enabling the body to respond more quickly to subsequent infections.

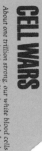

1 THE BATTLE BEGINS

As viruses begin to invade the body, a few are consumed by macrophages, which seize the antigens and display them on their own surfaces. Among millions of helper T cells circulating in the bloodstream, a select few are programmed to "read" that antigen. Binding to the macrophage, the T cell becomes activated.

2 THE FORCES MULTIPLY

Once activated, helper T cells begin to multiply. They then stimulate the multiplication of those few killer T cells and B cells that are sensitive to the invading viruses. As the number of B cells increases, helper T cells signal them to start producing antibodies.

3 CONQUERING THE INFECTION

Meanwhile, some of the viruses have entered cells of the body—the only place they are able to replicate. Killer T cells will sacrifice these cells by chemically puncturing their membranes, letting the contents spill out, thus disrupting the viral replication cycle. Antibodies then neutralize the viruses by binding directly to their surfaces, preventing them from attacking other cells. Additionally, they precipitate chemical reactions that actually destroy infected cells.

4 CALLING A TRUCE

As the infection is contained, suppressor T cells halt the entire range of immune responses, preventing them from spiraling out of control. Memory T and B cells are left in the blood and lymphatic system, ready to move quickly should the same virus once again invade the body.

A miracle of evolution, the human immune system is not controlled by any central organ, such as the brain. Rather it has developed to function as a kind of biologic democracy, wherein the individual members achieve their ends through an information network of awesome scope. Accounting for one percent of the body's 100 trillion cells, these defender white blood cells arise in the bone marrow. They fall into three groups: the phagocytes, or "cell eaters," of which the stalwart macrophage is one, and two kinds of lymphocytes, called T and B cells. All share one common objective: to identify and destroy all substances, living and inert, that are not part of the human body, that are "not self."

These include human cancer cells, which have turned from self to nonself, friend to foe.

There are four critical phases to each immune response: recognition of the enemy, amplification of defenses, attack, and slowdown. Each immune response is a unique local sequence of events, shaped by the nature of the enemies. Chemical toxins and a multitude of inert environmental substances, such as asbestos and smoke particles, are normally attacked only by phagocytes. Organic invaders enlist the full range of immune responses. Besides viruses, these include single-celled bacteria, protozoa, and fungi, as well as a host of multicelled worms called helminths. Many of these enemies have evolved devious methods to escape detection. The viruses that cause influenza and the common cold, for example, constantly mutate, changing their fingerprints. The AIDS virus, most insidious of all, employs a range of strategies, including hiding out in healthy cells. What makes it fatal is its ability to invade and kill helper T cells, thereby short-circuiting the entire immune response.

709

however, the viruses do not circulate in the bloodstream, and antibodies do not form. People, therefore, do not develop immunity to them. Antibodies *do* form to H.I.V. when it circulates in the bloodstream, but the H.I.V. antibodies are not capable of preventing H.I.V. from multiplying and doing its harm.

H.I.V. attacks the immune system by invading and destroying a particular type of white blood cell that scientists refer to by different names—you may hear it called the *helper T cell*, the T_4 *cell*, or the CD_4 *cell*. All these names refer to exactly the same kind of cell.

The helper T cell has also been informally dubbed the quarterback or field commander of the immune system. Helper T cells recognize invading pathogens and signal other white blood cells—called *B cells*—to produce antibodies that bind with pathogens. In binding with them, antibodies inactivate the pathogens and mark them for destruction. Helper T cells also signal another kind of T cell—the *killer T cell*—to destroy the cells that have been infected by the pathogen.

H.I.V. attacks helper T cells. By attacking and destroying helper T cells, H.I.V. disables the very cells that would allow the body to fight them and other disease-causing organisms off. As H.I.V. disables the immune system, the person becomes vulnerable to other infections and to forms of cancer that are normally held in check. Without an effective immune system, these diseases run out of control, eventually causing death.

The normal level of helper T cells in the circulatory system is about 1,000 per cubic millimeter of blood. During the first several years of H.I.V. infection, the numbers of helper T cells may stay at about this level. (People infected with H.I.V. tend not to look or act sick as long as the numbers of helper T cells remain high.) During the next five years or so of infection, however, the numbers of helper T cells may be chopped in half. Even so, many people still show no particular signs of illness. When the level of helper T cells falls below 200 per cubic millimeter of blood, however, people fall prey to a variety of illnesses.

COURSE OF H.I.V. INFECTION AND AIDS

Once in the body, H.I.V. follows a complex course of ups and downs—mostly downs. Many infected adults are symptom-free for years. In some people, however, H.I.V. may kill off large numbers of helper T cells shortly after infection. Such people are likely to have flulike symptoms such as fatigue, fever, headaches and muscle pain, poor appetite, nausea, swollen glands, and a rash. But the numbers of helper T cells then tend to rebound, such that these symptoms usually disappear within a few weeks. Most infected people then remain symptom-free for months or years. It is thus common for H.I.V.-infected people to think that they had a passing case of flu.

People who are infected with H.I.V. but symptom-free are said to be *carriers* of H.I.V. They are not yet obviously affected by H.I.V.

themselves, but they can transmit it to other people. Since they may not know that anything is wrong with them for many years, they can transmit H.I.V. to many other people without knowing what they are doing.

Some people who are infected with H.I.V., as noted, remain symptom-free carriers for many years. Others develop a cluster of symptoms (previously labeled *AIDS-related complex* or ARC) that includes chronic swollen lymph nodes, fatigue, fever, and periods of diarrhea and weight loss. These symptoms do not make up a 'full-blown' case of AIDS, but they indicate that H.I.V. is taking its toll on the immune system. People with such symptoms may still not recognize that they are infected with H.I.V. They may think that they are catching the 'things' that are going around—flu, colds, a stomach virus, whatever.

Perhaps ten or more years after the initial infection, H.I.V. begins to reproduce more rapidly. In the process, it destroys its host cells and spreads to infect other cells in the immune system. It eventually destroys the body's ability to fend off disease. Studies show that the average amount of time that passes between H.I.V. infection and development of a full-blown case of AIDS is about 10½ years.

AIDS is called a *syndrome* because it is characterized by a variety of symptoms. The beginnings of full-blown cases of AIDS are often marked by symptoms such as fatigue, night sweats, persistent fever, swollen lymph nodes, diarrhea, and unexplained weight loss. H.I.V. can also attack the central nervous system, causing *AIDS dementia complex* (or ADC). (Dementia is a state in which people are grossly confused and disorganized.) People with ADC show progressive losses in the abilities to concentrate, communicate, learn, remember things, understand what is happening around them, and control their muscle movements. More than half of people who develop AIDS eventually have such problems.

INDICATOR AND OPPORTUNISTIC DISEASES

People with AIDS are prone to developing certain diseases that are called *indicator diseases* or *opportunistic diseases*. These diseases include *Kaposi's sarcoma* (a rare form of cancer); *PCP* (a kind of pneumonia); parasitic infections of the brain (*toxoplasmosis*); herpes infections with chronic open sores; and what is called the 'wasting syndrome.'

The wasting syndrome literally involves wasting away. People with the syndrome lose weight without going on a diet or burning more calories through exercise. Indicator diseases are also known as opportunistic diseases because none of them is likely to take hold unless given the *opportunity* to do so by the weakening of the immune system.

WOMEN AND AIDS

Lily was not supposed to get AIDS. She was heiress to a cosmetics fortune. She had received her bachelor's degree from Wellesley and had been enrolled in a graduate program in art history when she came down with intractable flu-like symptoms and was eventually diagnosed as having AIDS.

'No one believed it,' she said. 'I was never a male homosexual in San Francisco. I never shot up crack in the alleys of The Bronx. My boyfriends didn't shoot up either. There was just Matthew . . .' Now Lily was 24. At 17, in her senior year in high school, she had had a brief affair with Matthew. Later she learned that Matthew was bisexual. Five years ago, Matthew died from AIDS.

'I haven't exactly been a whore,' Lily said ironically. 'You can count my boyfriends on the fingers of one hand.

None of them caught it from me; I guess I was just lucky.' Her face twisted in anger. 'You may think this is awful,' she said, 'but there are times when I wish Jerry and Russ had gotten it from me. Why should they get off?'

Lily's family was fully supportive, emotionally and, of course, financially. Lily had been to fine clinics. Physicians from Europe had been brought in. She was on a regimen of three medicines: two antiviral drugs, which singly and in combination held promise for slowing the progress of AIDS, and an antibiotic intended to prevent bacterial infections from taking hold. She took some vitamins—not megavitamin therapy. She exercised when she felt up to it, and she was doing reasonably well. In fact, there were times when she thought she might get over her illness.

'Sometimes I find myself thinking about children or grandchildren. Or sometimes I find myself looking at all these old pictures [of grandparents and other relatives] and thinking that I'll have silver in my hair, too. Sometimes I really think this is the day the doctors will call me about the new wonder drug that's been discovered in France or Germany.'

'I want to tell you about Russ,' she said once. 'After we found out about me, he went for testing, and he was clear [of antibodies indicative of infection by the AIDS virus]. He stayed with me, you know. When I wanted to do it, we used condoms. A couple of months later, he went for a second test and he was still clear. Then maybe he had second thoughts, because he became impotent—with me. We'd try, but he couldn't do anything. Still he stayed with me, but I felt us drifting apart. After a while, he was just doing the right thing by staying with me, and I'll

be damned if anyone is going to be with me because he's doing the right thing.'

Lily looked the [interviewer] in the eye. 'What sane man wants to play Russian roulette with AIDS for the sake of looking like a caring person? I'll tell you why I sent him away,' she added, tears welling. 'The one thing I've learned is that you die alone. I don't even feel that close to my parents anymore. Everyone loves you and wishes they could trade places with you, but they can't. You're suddenly older than everyone around you and you're going to go alone. I can't tell you how many times I thought about killing myself, just so that I could be the one who determines exactly where and when I die—how I would be dressed and how I would feel on the final day.'

Lily was suffering from AIDS—a syndrome that was unknown when she was born and was thought likely to affect only gay men and people who shoot up drugs when she was infected with H.I.V.

The number of women who have been struck by AIDS is on the rise. By 1987, AIDS had become one of the ten leading causes of death of American women of childbearing age (15 to 44). By 1991, AIDS had become one of the five leading causes of death of women in this age group. More than 15,000 U.S. women were diagnosed as having AIDS by the end of 1990. The incidence of AIDS is increasing more rapidly among women than men. Moreover, because women, like men, may be symptom-free for several years after they have been infected with H.I.V., the reported cases of women with AIDS may be only the tip of iceberg. According a Alexandra Levine,[1] an AIDS researcher at the University of Southern California:

We have not begun to see what's going to happen with women. We are now with women at the same situation we were for gay men in 1983 or 1984. It can happen to you or to me or to any of us. This is a sexually transmitted disease. Period. You must think of yourself as potentially at risk. It's the only way we're going to get on top of this epidemic.

Women now account for about 12 percent of AIDS cases in the United States, but for nearly one-third of the cases around the world. According to the U.S. Surgeon General Antonia Novello, nearly half of all cases of AIDS worldwide by the year 2000 will be among women. Approximately one in four women with AIDS is 20 to 29 years old, which suggests that many of them were infected as teenagers.

Lily was from a wealthy family. The risks of H.I.V. infection and the deaths associated with AIDS fall most heavily on poor African-American and Hispanic-American women who live in inner cities, however.

There are many questions about how H.I.V. infection and AIDS affect women. Much of our knowledge about the course of the illness derives from studies of homosexual men. It is not known whether the disease follows the same course in women. AIDS may have symptoms that go unrecognized or are misdiagnosed in women. Most drug trials have also been conducted on men, not on women or children, so questions remain about the effectiveness of antiviral drugs on women and children.

It is known that women AIDS patients are likely to develop a number of conditions that are not seen in men. 'Indicator diseases' that may be linked to H.I.V. infection and AIDS in women include *pelvic inflammatory disease* (or PID), *vaginal candidiasis*, and *precancerous cervical disease* (see Figure 3.2).

The symptoms of PID include abdominal pain or cramps, tenderness around the abdomen or cervix, nausea, vomiting, fever, cervical discharge, irregular menstrual cycles, and pain during sexual intercourse. Candidiasis is also known as a *yeast infection*. Candidiasis usually produces soreness, inflammation, and intense itching in the genital region that is accompanied by a white, thick, curdy vaginal discharge.

The *cervix* is the passageway between the vagina and the uterus. After sexual intercourse, semen passes through the cervix and uterus into the Fallopian tubes, where conception normally takes place. When a baby is born, it passes from the uterus through the cervix and the vagina to the outer world. Much of the pain of labor is caused by the stretching and thinning of the cervix. Cervical cancer is a common killer of women. In *precancerous* cervical disease, the cells in the cervix begin to change to cancerous cells.

These diseases—especially P.I.D. and yeast infections—are also found among many women who are *not* infected with H.I.V., however. Most of the time, their presence does *not* mean that the woman is infected with H.I.V. or has AIDS. Women should nevertheless report symptoms such as we have discussed to their doctors. Young women—especially sexually active young women—should also visit their gynecologists regularly so that the health of their outer and inner genital organs, including the cervix, can be evaluated.

Women apparently die faster of AIDS than men do. Women survive an average of seven months, as compared with two years for men. The reasons for this difference are not well understood, but researchers suspect that delayed intervention and treatment of women with AIDS may play a role.[2]

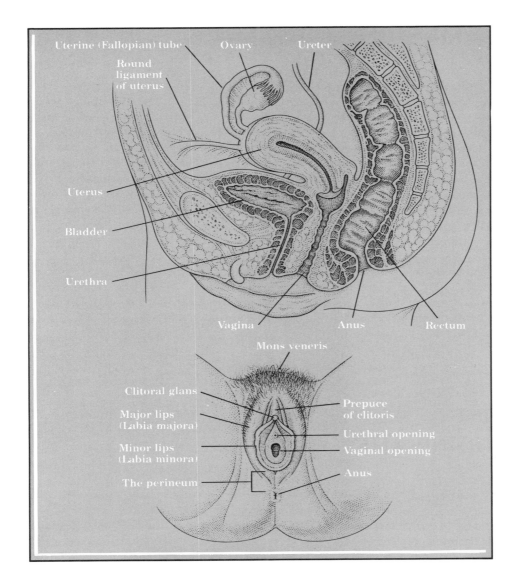

Uterine (Fallopian) tube Ovary Ureter

Round
ligament
of uterus

Uterus

Bladder

Urethra

Vagina Anus Rectum

Mons veneris

Clitoral glans

Major lips
(Labia majora)

Minor lips
(Labia minora)

The perineum

Prepuce
of clitoris

Urethral opening

Vaginal opening

Anus

Figure 3.2. Female Sexual Anatomy. The above drawing is a cross-section of the internal female reproductive organs. Some women who are infected with H.I.V. have precancerous changes in the cervix—the passageway between the vagina and uterus. Many sexually transmitted disease-causing organisms travel through the urethra to infect the bladder. The lower drawing provides a view of the external female reproductive organs (collectively termed the vulva). Symptoms of a number of sexually transmitted diseases, such as sores, are found on the vulva.

CHILDREN AND AIDS

Most babies who are infected with H.I.V. by their mothers during pregnancy appear normal at birth. They usually develop AIDS-related symptoms by six months of age, however. Full-blown cases of AIDS have usually developed by their second birthdays. Half of the babies who are infected with H.I.V. die of AIDS before their third birthdays.[3] H.I.V. infection in children differs from infection in adults in many ways. In infants, AIDS leads to bacterial infections and lung diseases that are not found in adults. H.I.V. directly infects infants' central nervous systems—that is, their brains and spinal cords. As a result, the children do not show normal growth patterns and are sometimes mentally retarded as well.

The kinds of opportunistic diseases that plague adults, such as Kaposi's sarcoma, are not usually found in children. The outcome is just as lethal, however. AIDS has become the ninth leading cause of death in children. If the trend in place continues, AIDS may become the leading cause of death in children! Boys and girls account for roughly equal numbers of cases of children with AIDS: 54 percent of cases are found among boys, and 46 percent are found among girls. The racial distribution is unequal, however. White people in the United States greatly outnumber African-Americans and Hispanic-Americans. As of the fall of 1991, however, 54 percent of the 3,312 AIDS cases among children were among African-American children; 24 percent were among Hispanic-American children; and only 21 percent were among white children.[4]

ADJUSTMENT OF PEOPLE WITH H.I.V. INFECTIONS AND AIDS

AIDS patients—men, women, and children—die from one or another opportunistic disease within a few years. After the onset of AIDS, the average length of survival for women and men combined is little more than a year. (Remember that H.I.V. and AIDS are not the same thing. It takes an average of 10½ years for people who are infected with H.I.V. to develop AIDS. Once they have developed AIDS, they can be expected to survive for another year or so.) A study of AIDS patients in San Francisco from 1981 to 1987 found that only 3 to 4 percent survived for five years. How do people respond when they learn that they are infected with H.I.V. and face such prospects?

AIDS victims often suffer psychological problems, most notably anxiety, depression, guilt about sexual behavior or drug abuse, anger, and—as in the case of Lily—suicidal feelings. People who are infected with H.I.V. are often angry with the medical profession for its failure to discover a cure or a vaccine for AIDS. They also tend to be angry with the public at large for discriminating against AIDS victims and not spending enough on the medical assault on AIDS. Many people are compassionate and supportive of AIDS victims, of course, but others are openly hostile or subtly rejecting. Many H.I.V./AIDS victims encounter discrimination in housing or employment. Children with H.I.V. infections or AIDS may be avoided in school and shunned by neighbors and their children.

When people learn that they are infected with H.I.V., they may at first deny the seriousness of the problem. Magic Johnson earned the title of most valuable player in an NBA all-star game after his infection was revealed. If an infected person can effectively battle athletes who are nearly seven feet tall, why worry about H.I.V. infection, one might ask? *Because in at least 99 percent of cases, people who are infected with H.I.V. will develop AIDS and die from it.*

For other people, the uncertainty of living with H.I.V. and the potential of developing AIDS often cause feelings of anxiety and depression.

Infected people are often preoccupied with fear of death, feelings of guilt about the behavior that led to the infection, and feelings of alienation from other people. As Lily said, when you die, you die alone. Stress weakens the immune system. The immune systems of infected people, which have already been weakened by H.I.V., may thus be further weakened by the stress caused by awareness of the infection. Many people with H.I.V. infections and AIDS have also lost friends or lovers to the disease. The stress imposed by these losses may further weaken their immune systems.

4 Transmission, Diagnosis, and Treatment of H.I.V. Infection and AIDS

Melanie is 18 years old and she lives in Massachusetts. She shares some concerns about AIDS—and how you talk about AIDS with someone you care about—with many young people today:

> How to bring up AIDS with someone you'd like to sleep with confuses me. I mean, what do you say? 'Gee, honey, I love you and want to have sex with you, but can you please take an AIDS test today and then lock yourself up for six months so I'm sure you won't sleep with anyone else and then take the test again? Then maybe I'll sleep with you.'[1]

In this chapter we discuss the transmission, diagnosis, and treatment of H.I.V. infection and AIDS. You will learn the different ways in which people have become infected with H.I.V., and you will see why Melanie was wondering whether or not she could ask a boyfriend to be tested, lock himself up for six months, and then be tested again.

TRANSMISSION OF H.I.V.

H.I.V. is transmitted through the blood, semen, and vaginal fluids of infected people. People come into contact with these fluids through vaginal and anal intercourse (anal intercourse—inserting the penis in the rectum—is a way in which male homosexuals have been infected), transfusions with contaminated blood (which is how tennis player and Wimbledon champion Arthur Ashe said he was infected[2]), transplants of infected organs and tissues, sharing hypodermic needles (as is common among people who inject or 'shoot up' drugs), or being stuck accidentally by a needle that was used on an infected person (which sometimes happens to health professionals such as nurses).

There is also some evidence that H.I.V. may be transmitted by oral sex with an infected partner, whether the partner is female or male, or through kissing in which saliva is exchanged. Deep tongue kissing (also referred to as French kissing or soul kissing) may carry a risk of infection because H.I.V. may be able to enter the bloodstream through cuts or sores in the lining of the mouth or gums. *You cannot transmit, or be infected with, H.I.V. sexually, however, if neither you nor your partner is infected, regardless of what you and your partner do.* H.I.V. may also be transmitted from mother to baby during pregnancy or through childbirth or breast-feeding.

It is more common for men to transmit H.I.V. to women through sexual intercourse than for women to transmit it to men in this way. One reason for the difference is that larger amounts of H.I.V. are found in semen than in vaginal fluids. Another reason is that infected semen may remain in the vagina for several days after a couple have engaged in sexual relations, thus providing a greater opportunity for infection. It also seems that cells in the cervix are particularly vulnerable to H.I.V. infection. Although women are at greater risk than men to be infected with H.I.V. through sexual intercourse, remember that Magic Johnson claimed to be infected by a woman.

Anal intercourse is considered to be an especially risky practice, particularly to the person who receives the penis in the rectum. The penis often scrapes or tears the inner lining of the rectum, making it easier for the H.I.V. in infected semen to enter the bloodstream.

Heterosexual (man-to-woman and woman-to-man) transmission, through sexual intercourse, is the primary route of H.I.V. infection in much of Africa, the Caribbean, and some parts of South America. Although more homosexuals than heterosexuals are infected with H.I.V. in the United States, heterosexual intercourse accounts for 75 percent of cases of H.I.V. infection worldwide. The number of cases of heterosexual transmission of H.I.V. has also been rising rapidly in the United States and Canada. This surge has raised concerns that H.I.V. and AIDS will spread widely into the general population through heterosexual sex.

Some women in the United States have contracted H.I.V. from heterosexual men who did not abuse drugs. We do not hear too much about them, however. When Magic Johnson announced his infection by H.I.V., for example, he noted that

in his travels as a basketball player, 'I was never at a loss for female companionship.'[3] He estimated that he had sexual relations with 2,000 women. Perhaps because of sexism, however; perhaps because of the forthright way in which Magic Johnson announced his infection; and perhaps because of Johnson's hero status, one newspaper reporter noted that 'There has been little public comment about the presumably innumerable women Johnson unknowingly placed in jeopardy.'[4]

In the early 1980s, H.I.V. spread rapidly among *hemophiliacs* who received contaminated blood in transfusions. Hemophiliacs lack clotting factors in the blood. They can thus bleed profusely when they are injured, and blood transfusions may be needed to replace lost blood. More than half of the nation's 20,000 hemophiliacs were infected with H.I.V. in the early years of the AIDS epidemic. In the mid-1980s, the test to detect H.I.V. antibodies (revealing the presence of H.I.V. infection) became available, and blood banks began screening blood donations. Since 1987, no hemophiliac in the United States is known to have contracted H.I.V. from a transfusion. Although a remote possibility of being infected with H.I.V. from blood transfusions continues to exist, people cannot be infected with H.I.V. by donating blood because the needles are used only once.

Ways in Which H.I.V. Is *Not* Transmitted

It is also important to understand the ways in which H.I.V. is *not* transmitted. Such knowledge will help set aside groundless concerns, such as needless fear of people who have been infected with H.I.V. It turns out that H.I.V. is *not* transmitted through casual contact such as handshakes, hugs, or jostling in a bus or train. H.I.V. is not transmitted by insect or mosquito bites. (H.I.V. cannot survive in the bloodstreams of insects.) Nor is H.I.V. transmitted by trying on clothes in a store; by handling doorknobs, money, or other objects used by infected people; or by sharing telephones, bathroom facilities, drinking fountains, or swimming pools with infected people. H.I.V. is not transmitted by contact with airborne germs or contaminated food, either. Nor is there evidence of transmission between infected persons and family members with whom they share food, eating utensils, toilet seats, or toothbrushes. Nor has it ever been shown that children are infected with H.I.V. by nonsexual contact with classmates, or that workers are infected by nonsexual contact with co-workers.

H.I.V. and Health-Care Workers

Only one known case of H.I.V. transmission from health care workers to patients has been reported. It involved a Florida dentist who died of AIDS after practicing for several years after being infected with H.I.V.[5] It is speculated that the dentist may have bled from a cut on his hand or used instruments that had punctured his skin or that were not sterilized after being used on an infected patient. Kimberly Bergalis, one of the patients who was believed to have contracted H.I.V. from the dentist, became a symbol of the public debate over the testing of health-care providers for H.I.V. infection before she succumbed to AIDS in 1991.

Health-care workers also face a risk of infection from accidental needle-sticks from needles used previously on infected patients. At least 40 health-care workers have been infected in this way.

Why Are Some People More Vulnerable to H.I.V. Infection Than Others?

One of the mysteries of H.I.V. transmission is that there is no clear connection between the number of times a person has sexual relations with an infected partner and the likelihood of transmission. The risk of transmission generally increases with the number of times one has sex, but some people seem to be more likely to transmit the virus than others, and some people seem to be especially vulnerable to infection. Some people become infected by a single sexual encounter with an infected person; others do not become infected by years of sex with an infected partner.

Studies in Africa, Europe, and the United States suggest that infection with *other* sexually transmitted diseases (STDs) may play a role in one's vulnerability to infection with H.I.V.[6] Some STDs such as syphilis and genital herpes produce open sores in the genital region. These sores may provide a port of entry for H.I.V. into the bloodstream. Other STDs such as gonorrhea, chlamydial infections, trichomoniasis, and genital warts inflame (redden) the genital region. Inflammation may heighten the risk of infection by bringing more blood into the region.

Other factors that may affect the risk of transmission include the amount of H.I.V. in the semen, one's sexual behavior, and circumcision. Researchers suspect that the amount of virus in semen may ebb and flow, peaking both early and later in the course of the infection. Sexual practices such as anal intercourse may provide easy access for the virus because of abrasions or tears in the rectal lining.

Circumcision is a procedure during which the foreskin of the penis is removed. Some people such as Jews perform routine circumcisions for religious reasons. Other groups circumcise male babies for health reasons. Uncircumcised men may be at higher risk of infection both because they tend to have more sores on the penis and because the virus tends to linger in the folds of the foreskin.[7] Certain cells in the foreskin may also be especially susceptible to H.I.V. infection.

People Who Have Been Especially Hard Hit by the AIDS Epidemic

People who have been particularly hard hit by the AIDS epidemic include homosexual men, people who inject drugs, their sex partners, hemophiliacs, and children born to infected women.

Homosexuals. In the United States, AIDS first struck the homosexual (gay) male community and was largely spread through anal sex (inserting the penis in the rectum). The homosexual male communities in San Francisco and New York were hit especially hard by the AIDS epidemic in the 1980s. Gay men still account for about half of the reported cases of AIDS in the United States. In recent years, however, the rate of infection among homosexuals has declined. The decrease has been largely attributed to increased use of safer sexual practices, including use of condoms, among gay men.

Only a handful of cases of the sexual transmission of H.I.V. from woman to woman have been reported. The women are assumed to transmit H.I.V. through oral sex or deep kissing, although the modes of transmission remain somewhat speculative.

People Who Inject ('Shoot Up') Drugs. At the same time that the incidence of new cases of AIDS has been declining among gay men, the rate of infection has been increasing among people who inject drugs (the majority of whom are men) and their sex partners (the majority of whom are women). People who inject drugs account for about one AIDS case in four in the United States. The drugs that are most likely to be injected are cocaine and heroin. As you can see in Table 4.1, however, these drugs are not particularly popular on college campuses.

Alcohol is the most popular drug on high school and college campuses, and alcohol, of course, is drunk, not injected. Table 4.1 shows a ten-year trend for college students, according to University of Michigan surveys. Note that overall drug use at college has declined in recent years.

Drug abuse is generally higher among African-, Hispanic-, and Native-American adolescents than among white adolescents. The extent of drug abuse also depends on where these adolescents live, and whether or not they drop out of school. The highest rates of abuse occur where poor minority group members live in segregated neighborhoods. For example, African-Americans who live in the 'ghetto,' Hispanic-Americans who dwell in the barrio, and Native Americans who live on the reservation all have high rates of drug abuse. Adolescents who live in such neighborhoods are more likely to encounter social isolation, unemployment, poverty, and deviant role models, some of whom are gang members. People from these ethnic groups who attend college are relatively less likely to abuse drugs and to be infected with H.I.V.

The adolescents who are at greatest risk for drug abuse and H.I.V. infection through sharing contaminated needles also tend to drop out of school. For this reason, school-based surveys tend to underestimate drug abuse by minority groups. The national high-school drop-out rate is about 27 percent, and inner-city adolescents with the worst crime and drug problems are not included in such surveys, so their numbers remain unknown.

About half of the American women who have AIDS were apparently infected with H.I.V. through the use of contaminated hypodermic needles. About three women victims in four live in large metropolitan areas, often in impoverished inner cities.

H.I.V. infection appears to be higher among women who use cocaine. In some cases the women inject cocaine. Even women who take cocaine in other ways are more likely to engage in risky sexual behavior, such as prostitution or unprotected intercourse with men who inject drugs, than are women who do not use cocaine.

Table 4.1
PERCENTAGE OF COLLEGE STUDENTS WHO REPORT DRUG USE
'DURING THE LAST 30 DAYS,' 1981–1991

Drug	1981	1982	1983	1984	1985	1986	1987	1988	1989	1990	1991
Alcohol	81.9	82.8	80.3	79.1	80.3	79.7	78.4	77.0	76.2	74.5	74.7
Cigarettes	25.9	24.4	24.7	21.5	22.4	22.4	24.0	22.6	21.1	21.5	23.2
Marijuana	33.2	26.8	26.2	23.0	23.6	22.3	20.3	16.8	16.3	14.0	14.1
Cocaine	7.3	7.9	6.5	7.6	6.9	7.0	4.6	4.2	2.8	1.2	1.0
(Crack)	NA*	NA	NA	NA	NA	NA	0.4	0.5	0.2	0.1	0.3
Other stimulants	12.3	9.9	7.0	5.5	4.2	3.7	2.3	1.8	1.3	1.4	1.0
Sedatives Barbiturates, Methaqualone	3.4	2.5	1.1	1.0	0.7	0.6	0.6	0.6	0.2	0.2	0.3
Hallucinogens	2.3	2.6	1.8	1.8	1.3	2.2	2.0	1.7	2.3	1.4	1.2
Heroin	0.0	0.0	0.0	0.0	0.0	0.0	0.1	0.1	0.1	0.0	0.1

*NA = Not available.
Source of table: Johnston, L. D., Bachman, J. G., & O'Malley, P. M. (1992, January 25). Monitoring the future: A continuing study of the lifestyles and values of youth. The University of Michigan News and Information Services: Ann Arbor, MI.

Infants Born to Sex Partners of People Who Inject Drugs. In New York City, for example, the majority of children who are born infected with the H.I.V. virus have mothers who inject drugs or whose sex partners do.

Prostitutes. Prostitutes who abuse drugs or who engage in unprotected sex with clients or people who inject drugs are at particular risk. In some locations, such as Newark, New Jersey and Miami, Florida, nearly half of the street prostitutes are infected with H.I.V.

Men Who Frequent Prostitutes. No one knows how many people in the United States engage in prostitution or frequent prostitutes. In the nineteenth-century United States, married and unmarried men visited prostitutes regularly, and young men were often initiated into sexual activity by prostitutes. It was common, even expected, for young men to 'sow their wild oats' with prostitutes. Surveys of young men today, however, show that only a small minority of men are sexually initiated by prostitutes. Contemporary couples are relatively less likely to demand virginity in brides, so young men today are much more likely to become sexually initiated with their girlfriends than by prostitutes. Concerns about the spread of sexually transmitted diseases, especially AIDS, have also contributed to the decline in the use of prostitutes.

Sex with prostitutes is considered the most important factor in the heterosexual transmission of H.I.V. in Africa, where H.I.V. is spread predominantly by means of heterosexual intercourse.[8] A Florida study showed that regular contact with female street prostitutes was also a risk factor in the transmission of H.I.V. in American men.[9] Prostitutes are at risk of being infected by H.I.V. because they have sexual relations with many partners, often without condoms. Moreover, many prostitutes and their sex partners shoot up drugs and share contaminated needles.[10]

Sex Partners of Men Who Frequent Prostitutes.
H.I.V. may be spread by unprotected sex from prostitutes to customers, and then to the customers' wives or lovers.

Estimating Your Own Risk of Being Infected by H.I.V.

Many groups of people have thus been hit especially hard by the AIDS epidemic. Bear in mind, however, that it is people's behavior, and not the groups to which they belong, that determines whether or not they are at risk of being infected with H.I.V. Table 4.2 estimates the risk of being infected by sex partners who do or do not belong to groups that have been particularly hard hit by the AIDS epidemic.

Let's do some frank talking about Table 4.2—about what it suggests and does not suggest to readers. Overall, the table might give you the impression that as a student you have little to worry about. After all, you might think, there's no 'real' chance that your partner is gay, injects drugs, belongs to any other hard-hit group, or is seropositive. It might thus seem to you that your

chances of being infected by H.I.V. are less than one in a million or even less than one in a billion. True? Not necessarily!

First of all, the great (great!) majority of people you know and date will fall into the category of 'serostatus unknown.' That means that they will not have been tested for H.I.V. infection. If the person you are thinking of is heterosexual, it is also unlikely that she or he will fall into any of the known risk groups. As noted in Table 4.1, for example, only a small minority of college students report using drugs of the sort that are injected.

Alcohol is the most commonly used drug among college students, and you might assume that you cannot be infected by H.I.V. by drinking alcohol. Technically, of course, you do not become infected by drinking alcohol, or even by sharing beverages with an infected person. The great majority of college students drink, however, and many of them admit to doing things when drunk that they would not do when sober—such as driving recklessly, engaging in unprotected sex, or having sexual relations with someone they would otherwise refuse. In fact, 20 to 25 percent of the students surveyed at the University of Virginia admitted to engaging in 'unwise' sexual relations under the influence of alcohol.[11]

Look again at Table 4.2. When your partner's serostatus is unknown, he or she may belong to a high-risk group and not tell you about it. What, for example, if you partner is *bisexual* rather than heterosexual and has (or did have) another sex life that you are unaware of? What if your partner is heterosexual but had a number of homosexual experiences in high school? What if your partner used to inject drugs but hasn't told you about it, or has lied about it?

Would fellow students lie to you about whether or not they are infected with H.I.V.? According to a poll of 18- to 25-year-old college students, they might do just that.[12] As you can see in Table 4.3, many college students admit to lying to their current sex partners, or else confess that they would if it were necessary. Many more college men admit to lying than college women do, and

Table 4.2
THE RISK OF BECOMING INFECTED WITH H.I.V. AS A RESULT OF HETEROSEXUAL INTERCOURSE

RISK CATEGORY OF PARTNER	Estimated Risk of Infection	
	ONE ACT OF INTERCOURSE	500 ACTS OF INTERCOURSE

H.I.V. serostatus* unknown

Partner Is Not in Any High-Risk Group[†]

Using latex condoms	1 in 50,000,000	1 in 110,000
Not using latex condoms	1 in 5,000,000	1 in 16,000

Partner Is in a High-Risk Group

Using latex condoms	1 in 10,000	1 in 21
Not using latex condoms	1 in 1,000	1 in 3

H.I.V. seronegative

Partner Has No History of High-Risk Behavior[†]

Using latex condoms	1 in 5,000,000,000	1 in 11,000,000
Not using latex condoms	1 in 500,000,000	1 in 1,600,000

Partner Currently Engages in High-Risk Behavior

Using latex condoms	1 in 500,000	1 in 1,100
Not using latex condoms	1 in 50,000	1 in 160

H.I.V. seropositive

Using latex condoms	1 in 5,000	1 in 11
Not using latex condoms	1 in 500	2 in 3

Serostatus, or 'blood status,' refers to the results of a blood test for H.I.V. antibodies. People whose results are seropositive have H.I.V. antibodies in their bloodstreams. People whose results are seronegative did not show H.I.V. antibodies in their bloodstreams. (If they have been infected with H.I.V. recently, however, H.I.V. antibodies may not develop and become evident within a few weeks or months. People who have reason to suspect that they may have been infected may thus desire to have repeated tests.)

[†]High-risk *groups* include gay men, people who inject drugs, sex partners of people who inject drugs, and hemophiliacs. High-risk *behaviors* include sexual activity or needle sharing with a member of one of these groups.

Source: Table adapted from Hearst, N., & Hulley, S. B. (1988). Preventing the heterosexual spread of AIDS: Are we giving our patients the best advice? *Journal of the American Medical Association, 259,* 2428–2432.

Table 4.3

PERCENTAGE OF COLLEGE STUDENTS (AGES 18–25) WHO SAY THEY *HAVE* LIED, OR *WOULD* LIE, TO SOMEONE TO PERSUADE HIM OR HER TO HAVE SEX

	Men	Women
Have you ever told anyone a lie in order to persuade him or her to engage in sexual activity?	34%	10%
Have you ever lied about your ejaculatory control? (Have you said you could safely engage in sexual activity without 'coming'?)	38	—
Have you ever lied about the likelihood of your getting pregnant?	—	14
Have you ever been sexually involved with more than one person at the same time?	32	23
If you were sexually involved with more than one person at the same time, did you keep your sex partners in the dark about it?	68	59
Have you ever been lied to by anyone who wanted to have sex with you?	47	60
Did your sex partner ever lie to you about his ability to control ejaculation? (Did he ever lie to you that you didn't have to worry about his 'coming' when there was good reason to worry?)	—	46
Did your sex partner ever lie to you about the likelihood of her getting pregnant?	34	—
Would you lie to someone and say you had a negative H.I.V.-antibody test in order to persuade him or her to have sex, when, in fact, you were not tested or had tested positive?	20	4
Would you lie to someone and say that you had fewer sex partners in the past than you really had in order to talk him or her into having sex?	47	42
Would you disclose the existence of another sex partner to a new sex partner?		
Never	22	10
After a while, when it was safe to tell him or her	34	28
Only if asked about it	31	33
Yes	13	29
Would you disclose a single episode of sexual infidelity to a steady date, a fiancé, or a spouse?		
Never	43	34
After a while, when it was safe to tell him or her	21	20
Only if asked about it	14	11
Yes	22	35

Source: Adapted from Cochran, S. D., & Mays, V. M. (1990). Sex, lies, and H.I.V. *The New England Journal of Medicine, 322,* 774–775. (Based on a sample of 196 college men and 226 college women.)

more college women say that they have been lied to by their sex partners. The message seems clear: Many students (just like many people who are not students!) will say or do what they have to do to get into bed with you. We are not saying that students as a group are not to be trusted. We *are* saying that many students admit to lying to their sex partners. You could be one of those partners, especially if you are a woman.

Table 4.2 also provides a good deal of information that fits with common sense. The more times you engage in sexual intercourse with an H.I.V.-infected partner, for example, the more likely you are to become infected with H.I.V. yourself.

If you have an ongoing sexual relationship with a partner who belongs to a group who has been hard hit by the epidemic, don't be complaisant about it because you're on the pill. Your chances of becoming infected are estimated to be about one in three. (The birth-control pill may prevent you from becoming pregnant, but it confers *no* protection against H.I.V. infection.) If you have an ongoing sexual relationship with a partner who not only belongs to a high-risk group but also happens to be infected, your own chances of becoming infected are estimated at about two in three. Even if you consistently use latex condoms, your chances of being infected by a continuing sexual relationship with a partner who tests positive for H.I.V. infection are about one in eleven.

DIAGNOSIS

What if you are wondering whether or not you or your partner has been infected with H.I.V.? How can you find out?

H.I.V. infection can be diagnosed by a blood test called ELISA, which is short for *enzyme-linked immunosorbent assay*. ELISA detects the presence of H.I.V. *antibodies* in the bloodstream. People typically develop antibodies to H.I.V. infection long before they develop any symptoms of infection, and many years before they develop AIDS.[13] Although the antibody test does not directly reveal the presence of the virus, a positive (seropositive) test result usually[14] indicates that the person has been infected with H.I.V. and that the body's immune system has produced antibodies against it. A negative result (seronegative) indicates that antibodies have not been found. Table 4.4 shows the prevalences of seropositive test results among various populations.

A more sophisticated blood test—the Western blot test—can be performed for persons who test seropositive to help ensure that the initial results were accurate. The Western blot test looks for a specific pattern of protein bands that are associated with the virus.

Since it may take months—now and then, a year or more—for antibodies to develop in people who have been infected with H.I.V., repeated tests may be advisable. Efforts are under way to develop less expensive and more accurate tests.

The presence of H.I.V. antibodies does not indicate whether, or when, an H.I.V.-infected person will develop AIDS. The diagnosis of AIDS has traditionally required the appearance of certain so-called indicator diseases, such as Kaposi's sarcoma or PCP, in a person who was seropositive for H.I.V. The Federal Centers for Disease Control (CDC) may extend the definition of AIDS to include people whose number of helper T cells have fallen below 200 per cubic millimeter of blood. Such an extended definition of AIDS would apply more equally to men, women, and children, so that more people would qualify for medical and other AIDS-related benefits. The redefinition would also increase the numbers of people who are diagnosed with AIDS.

Table 4.4
PREVALENCES OF POSITIVE RESULTS TO H.I.V. TESTING

Groups revealing low rates of infection (less than 0.1%)	Blood donors Military recruits and personnel Couples seeking marriage licenses
Groups at higher risk (positive results between 1% and 5%)	Prostitutes Patients with other sexually transmitted diseases (STDs) Babies born in New York City
Groups showing the highest rates of infection (prevalences of positive results as high as 50% to 80%)	Hemophiliacs receiving clotting factors People who inject ('shoot up') drugs and share needles while doing so Sexually active gay men

Source of data: Jacobsen, P. B., Perry, S. W., & Hirsch, D. (1990). Behavioral and psychological responses to HIV antibody testing. *Journal of Consulting and Clinical Psychology, 58,* 31–37.

Issues Concerning Testing for H.I.V.

Testing for H.I.V. antibodies is widely available, but there is no rush on the medical facilities that offer testing. Being tested for H.I.V. antibodies is not a simple issue. Consider the following thoughts that some young people share about testing:[15]

> A boyfriend of mine got very angry with me when he wanted to have sex without a condom and I wouldn't let him. He was quite promiscuous, and how should I know how clean those other women were? We both wanted to be tested for AIDS, but we didn't because we were too scared. If one of us did have AIDS, we really wouldn't know what to do.
> —Maureen, 19, Florida

> With my last boyfriend, we usually used a condom because we wanted to be safe.

> I took an AIDS test to get him to take one, but he never did. He was afraid of a false positive,[16] he said. Next time I will make the man take a test, unless he is a virgin.
> —Sharon, 21, Massachusetts

Attitudes toward testing vary. Some people, including some students, would not consider sexual relations with anyone who has not been tested and found to be seronegative. Some people even wait another six months or longer for a retesting. Other people do not request a partner to have a test for fear that the suggestion of a lack of trust will jeopardize the relationship. Some people have difficulty raising the subject of testing with their partners. Some people want to know their H.I.V. status so that they can assure their partners (and themselves!) that they are not infected with H.I.V.

Testing for H.I.V. infection raises important emotional, medical, ethical, and moral concerns. Some people argue that people have a moral obligation to learn about their H.I.V. status so that they can inform their sex partners and take appropriate safeguards, such as practicing safer sex, if necessary. Others argue that safer sex should be used regardless of one's H.I.V. status and that testing only stigmatizes people who are infected. Some people argue that H.I.V. testing is unnecessary for people who do not belong to the groups who have been hit hardest by the epidemic. Others argue that testing is just too risky for people—perhaps most of us—who might not be able to handle the emotional consequences of testing positive.

On the other hand, early diagnosis of H.I.V. infection may help relieve suffering and prolong life through the use of drugs that combat H.I.V. and the opportunistic infections that take hold in people with weakened immune systems. Even so, reports on the effectiveness of such drugs are mixed, and the drugs do not represent a cure for H.I.V. infection or AIDS.

Should You and Your Partner Be Tested for H.I.V.?

Readers who are debating whether or not they and their sex partners should be tested for H.I.V. may wish to weigh the following considerations:

1. *Is it likely that you are infected with H.I.V.?* Have you or a sex partner had sexual relations with a person at high risk of being infected? Have you shared needles with such a person? Do you feel a moral obligation to a sex partner to learn about your H.I.V. status?

2. *Are you prepared to handle news of a positive test result?* Could you cope with the emotional trauma of learning that you are infected?

3. *How might knowledge of your H.I.V. status affect your health?* Have you asked your physician whether early detection and intervention might benefit your health?

4. *If you learned that you were infected, would you really be able to inform a sex partner—or partners?*

5. *How would living with knowledge of being infected with H.I.V. affect your lifestyle?* How might such knowledge affect your education, your family life, your social relationships, and your sex life?

6. *How would you cope with possible public disclosure of your H.I.V. status?* About fifteen states now require that doctors, hospitals, and clinics that test for H.I.V. antibodies report the names of people who show positive test results. Reporting is intended to help state officials trace the sexual and needle-sharing contacts of infected people to alert them to the possibility of exposure to the virus. How would it affect you if health officials attempted to trace people whom you might have infected?

Notice that we're not suggesting an 'answer' as to whether you should be tested for H.I.V. Testing is voluntary today. That means that it is your decision. We have tried to enumerate some of the issues you might want to consider in making that decision.

TREATMENT

Unless a cure is found, I will be another one of your statistics soon. . . . I'm dying guys. Goodbye.
—Kimberly Bergalis[17]

Kimberly Bergalis died of AIDS in 1991. There have been too many Kimberlys, and there will be more.

Unfortunately, there is neither a cure for AIDS nor an effective, safe vaccine. As we write these pages, the outlook for a cure remains bleak. Some progress is reported in the effort to develop a vaccine. Several preparations have shown some success in animal trials and are now being tested in people. The extent of the tragedy of AIDS is underscored by the fact that AIDS patients are generally willing to try experimental vaccines and drugs. They see themselves as having little or nothing to lose. In any event, many researchers believe that a safe and effective vaccine will eventually be developed.

The antiviral drug *zidovudine* (formerly called azidothymidine, or AZT for short) has shown mixed results in treating AIDS patients and people who are infected with H.I.V. First, the promising news. Some studies have shown that zidovudine slows the progress of AIDS[18] and can delay the development of AIDS in people infected with H.I.V. who have not yet developed any AIDS-related symptoms.[19] Zidovudine seems to inhibit the ability of the H.I.V. virus to reproduce and appears to reduce the number of opportunistic infections. In one experimental trial, AIDS patients who received zidovudine survived an average of 770 days (about two years), as compared with 190 days (a bit more than half a year) among patients who did not receive the drug.[20]

Now, the negatives. Zidovudine can have serious side effects, including nausea, vomiting, diarrhea, a skin rash, and lowering of the number of lymphocytes in the bloodstream. Decreasing the numbers of lymphocytes further weakens the immune systems of people who are infected with H.I.V.

In 1991, a second drug—*dideoxyinosine* (DDI)—was approved for use in treating AIDS, even though it was still considered experimental. DDI is intended for people who have not been helped by zidovudine, cannot tolerate zidovudine, or develop resistance to it. DDI apparently increases the level of helper T cells in AIDS patients.

The approval of DDI signals the readiness of the Food and Drug Administration to speed the introduction of drugs which have the potential to help AIDS patients. Not all medical authorities believe that it is wise to rush a drug to market before careful tests of its safety and efficacy are conducted, however.

Researchers around the world are working on ways of treating people who are infected with H.I.V. Some are variations on existing themes. Some are quite different. In one experimental approach, for example, concentrated doses of H.I.V. antibodies kill the virus in the laboratory.[21] Infected people normally do not produce sufficient amounts of H.I.V. antibodies to eradicate H.I.V. in their bloodstreams. Time will tell whether it is possible to mass produce the needed antibodies and whether they actually do the job when they are injected into patients' bloodstreams.

People who are infected with H.I.V. may also be able to prolong their health by generally taking good care of themselves, getting enough sleep, avoiding unnecessary stress, eating a balanced diet, and avoiding becoming re-infected.

Despite all the medical details, the bottom line on H.I.V. today remains relatively clear and simple:

1. Certain behavior patterns place students (and other people) at risk of being infected with H.I.V.

2.　It is estimated that 99 percent or more of the people who are infected with H.I.V. will eventually develop AIDS, even if they have no symptoms of AIDS-related illnesses for many years.

3.　There is no effective and safe vaccine for H.I.V. infection or AIDS.

4.　Although there are many treatments for H.I.V. infection and AIDS, none of them is a cure.

People who are infected with H.I.V. are also likely to contract other sexually transmitted diseases (STDs). In the following chapter we discuss a number of them. In Chapter 6 we will discuss *prevention*—a term that has many meanings and has sparked much controversy.

AIDS Toll-Free Hotline Number: 1-800-342-AIDS

5

Other Sexually Transmitted Diseases

Because of its lethality, AIDS has been front-page news for a decade. Other sexually transmitted diseases (STDs) pose wider if less deadly threats, however. In Chapter 1 we reported on a study of 16,000 U.S. college students on nineteen campuses.[1] It was found that one student in 500 was infected with H.I.V. It was also found, however, that *chlamydia trachomatis* (the bacterium that causes chlamydia) and *human papilloma virus* (H.P.V.) (the virus that causes genital warts) were found in one student in ten. That's 10 percent of the college population! The same survey found that students were reasonably well informed about AIDS, but many students were unaware that chlamydia could go undetected for years, causing pelvic inflammation, scarring, and infertility. Many students had never even heard of H.P.V., *which is not to be confused with H.I.V.* H.P.V. is the virus that causes genital warts and has been linked to cervical cancer in women.

STDs are the most widespread communicable diseases in the United States. Nearly half of the Americans who are infected with STDs are younger than the age of 25. Some of you may have STDs today and not be aware of them. Others of you may be troubled by the symptoms of STDs, but you may not connect them to an STD. Ignorance is not bliss, however. Some STDs damage the internal reproductive system if they are left untreated—even when you are free of symptoms such as pain, itching, or discharges. Despite the threat imposed by STDs, many people find it difficult to raise the issue with their partners. One young woman explains that

it's one thing to talk about 'being responsible about STD' and a much harder thing to do it at the very moment. It's just plain hard to say to someone I am feeling very erotic with, 'Oh, yes, before we go any further, can we have a conversation about STD?' It's hard to imagine murmuring into someone's ear at a time of passion, 'Would you mind slipping on this condom or using this cream just in case one of us has an STD?' Yet it seems awkward to bring it up beforehand, if it's not yet clear between us that we want to make love with one another.[2]

Awkwardness is just one of the reasons that college students are reluctant to talk about STDs. Another is lack of knowledge about them—which we hope that this book is correcting. Still another is the 'heat of the moment.' Some people become so sexually aroused, especially when they are with a new partner, that caution flies to the winds and they risk unwanted pregnancies as well as STDs.

Because of the difficulties involved in talking about STDs with sex partners, many young people admit that they 'wing it.' They assume that their partners are free of STDs and hope for the best.

There is a surge today in the incidence of many STDs. One reason is the high number of young people who are engaging in sexual relations. Many people practice *unprotected sex*. (Sex with condoms ['rubbers,' 'safes'] is considered 'protected' sex.) Another reason is the widespread use of the birth-control pill. Birth-control pills are highly reliable methods of *contraception*—that is, if they are taken regularly, they will almost certainly prevent people from getting pregnant. Birth-control pills offer *no* protection against infection by organisms that cause STDs, however.

Still another reason for the rising incidence of STDs is the fact that some infections, like chlamydia, are often symptom-free. Infected individuals can thus unknowingly pass them along to others.

In this chapter, we discuss STDs that are caused by bacteria, viruses, and other pathogens.

STDs Caused by Bacteria

Bacteria are one-celled microorganisms that cause many illnesses, including strep throat, meningitis, and scarlet fever. They also give rise to the STDs of gonorrhea, syphilis, and chlamydia.

Gonorrhea

In a book with relatively little good news, let us start with a hopeful sign of progress in the fight against STDs. The rate of gonorrheal infection in the United States declined substantially during the 1980s. *Gonorrhea* (pronounced GONE-a-REE-a) nevertheless remains one of the most common STDs in the United States. Approximately three quarters of a million people in the United States contract gonorrhea each year. Many cases of gonorrhea go unreported, however, so the actual incidence may be as high as 3 million to 5 million cases per year. Most new cases of gonorrhea are contracted by young people between the ages of 20 and 24.

Gonorrhea—also known as 'the clap' or 'the drip'—is caused by the gonococcus bacterium (see Table 5.1). The gonococcus bacterium was isolated in 1879 and named after its discoverer, Albert L. S. Neisser: *Neisseria gonorrhoeae.*

Gonococcal bacteria thrive in a warm, moist environment, like that found along the mucus membranes of the urinary tract in men and women or of the cervix in women. Outside the body, they die quickly. Gonorrhea is almost always transmitted by unprotected vaginal, oral, or anal sexual activity. There is no evidence that gonorrhea can be caught from toilet seats or by touching dry objects.

The eyes provide a good environment for the bacterium. So if you handle the genitals of an infected person and then touch your eyes, you may infect them.

Most men experience symptoms within two to five days after infection. Symptoms include a discharge from the penis that is clear at first. Within a day, the discharge becomes yellow to yellow-green, thicker, and pus-like. The urethra (the passageway for urine) becomes inflamed, and it burns when men urinate. Many men have swelling and tenderness in the groin.

These symptoms often subside without treatment after a few weeks. Infected people may thus conclude, erroneously, that gonorrhea is no worse than a bad case of the 'flu.' Even when early symptoms subside, however, gonorrhea usually remains at work within the body.

In women the primary site of the infection is the cervix. It causes *cervicitis*—an inflammation of the cervix—which may be accompanied by a yellowish to yellow-green pus-like discharge that irritates the genital region. If the infection spreads to the urethra, women may also note burning urination. *About 80 percent of the women who contract gonorrhea have no symptoms during the early stages of the disease, however.* Unfortunately, they may not seek treatment until more serious symptoms develop.

Table 5.1

PATHOGENS, TRANSMISSION, SYMPTOMS, DIAGNOSIS,
AND TREATMENT OF MAJOR SEXUALLY TRANSMITTED DISEASES

PATHOGEN	TRANSMISSION	SYMPTOMS	DIAGNOSIS	TREATMENT
GONORRHEA ('clap,' 'drip'): Gonococcus bacterium (called *Neisseria gonorrhoeae*)	Vaginal, oral, or anal sexual activity, or from mother to baby during childbirth	In men, a yellowish, thick penile discharge and burning urination In women, an increased vaginal discharge, burning urination, irregular menstrual bleeding (most women are symptom-free in early stages of illness)	Culture of a sample of the discharge	Antibiotics such as ceftriaxone and spectinomycin
SYPHILIS: *Treponema pallidum* bacterium	Vaginal, oral, or anal sexual activity, or by touching an infectious chancre (sore)	A hard, round painless chancre appears at the site of the infection during the primary stage (within two to four weeks). Syphilis may progress through secondary, latent, and tertiary stages, if it is left untreated.	In the primary-stage, syphilis is diagnosed by clinical examination; fluid from a chancre may also be examined for the bacteria that cause the disease. The VDRL (a blood test) is used to diagnose secondary-stage syphilis.	Antibiotics such as penicillin, doxycycline, tetracycline, or erythromycin

Table 5.1, continued

PATHOGEN	TRANSMISSION	SYMPTOMS	DIAGNOSIS	TREATMENT
CHLAMYDIA and NONGONOCOCCAL URETHRITIS (NGU): *Chlamydia trachomatis* bacterium; NGU in men may also be caused by *Ureaplasma urealycticum* bacterium or other pathogens	Vaginal, oral, or anal sexual activity; babies may be infected by mothers during childbirth.	In women, urination may be frequent and painful; there may also be pain and inflammation in the lower abdomen and a vaginal discharge (but most women are symptom-free). In men, symptoms are similar to but milder than those of gonorrhea: burning or painful urination and a penile discharge (some men are asymptomatic) Infection through oral sex may cause a sore throat.	In women, a cervical smear is analyzed by the Abbott Testpack.	Antibiotics such as doxycycline, tetracycline, and erythromycin (penicillin is usually ineffective)
BACTERIAL VAGINOSIS: *Gardnerella vaginalis* bacterium and others	Sexual contact (may arise originally by overgrowth of organisms in the vagina, allergic reactions, and so on)	In women, there may be a thin, foul-smelling vaginal discharge, irritation of genitals, and mild pain during urination. In men, there may be inflammation of the foreskin and glans of the penis, urethritis, and cystitis.	Culture and examination of bacterium	Oral treatment with metronidazole (marketed as Flagyl)

PATHOGEN	TRANSMISSION	SYMPTOMS	DIAGNOSIS	TREATMENT
CANDIDIASIS (moniliasis, thrush, 'yeast infection'): *Candida albicans*—a yeastlike fungus	Sexual contact, or sharing a washcloth with an infected person (can arise originally by overgrowth of the fungus in the vagina).	In women, there may be vulval itching; a white, cheesy, foul-smelling discharge; soreness or swelling of vaginal and nearby tissues. In men, there may be itching and burning on urination, or a reddening of the penis.	Diagnosis is generally made on basis of symptoms.	Miconazole, clotrimazole, or teraconazole in the form of vaginal suppositories, creams or tablets; keeping the affected area dry
TRICHOMONIASIS ('trich'): *Trichomonas vaginalis*—a protozoan (one-celled animal)	Sexual activity	In women, there may be a foamy, yellowish, odorous, discharge and itching or burning sensations (many women are symptom-free). Men are usually asymptomatic, but there may be mild urethritis.	Microscopic examination of a smear of vaginal secretions, or of culture of the smear	Metronidazole (Flagyl)
ORAL HERPES: *Herpes simplex virus-type 1 (H.S.V.-1)*	Sexual contact with sores or blisters; touching, kissing; sharing cups, towels, toilet seats	Cold sores or fever blisters on the lips, mouth, or throat; on the genitals, symptoms take the form of herpetic sores.	Usually by clinical inspection	Nonprescription lip balms and cold-sore medications (Be certain of the diagnosis before you treat yourself, however.)

PATHOGEN	TRANSMISSION	SYMPTOMS	DIAGNOSIS	TREATMENT
GENITAL HERPES: *Herpes simplex virus-type 2 (H.S.V.-2)*	Vaginal, oral, or anal sexual activity (People are most contagious during active outbreaks of the disease.)	Painful, reddish bumps around the genitals, thigh, or buttocks (In women, the bumps may also be found in the vagina or on the cervix.) The bumps become blisters or sores that fill with pus and break, shedding viral particles. There may also be burning urination, fever, aches and pains, swollen glands, and—in women—a vaginal discharge.	Clinical inspection of sores; culture and examination of fluid drawn from the base of a sore	The antiviral drug acyclovir (marketed as Zovirax) may offer relief and promote healing but is not a cure.
HEPATITIS: Hepatitis A-, B-, C-, and D-type viruses	Sexual contact, especially involving the anus; contact with infected fecal matter; transfusion of contaminated blood	There may be flu-like symptoms including fever, abdominal pain, vomiting, and jaundiced (yellowish) skin and eyes. (Some people with hepatitis are asymptomatic.)	Examination of blood for hepatitis antibodies	Bed rest, fluids (and sometimes antibiotics to ward off other infections that might take hold because of lowered resistance.)

PATHOGEN	TRANSMISSION	SYMPTOMS	DIAGNOSIS	TREATMENT
GENITAL WARTS (venereal warts): *Human papilloma virus (H.P.V.)*	Sexual and other forms of contact, as with infected towels or clothing	Painless warts that may resemble cauliflowers on the penis, scrotum, or urethra in men, and on the vulva, labia, vaginal wall, or cervix in women. May also be found around the anus and in the rectum.	Clinical inspection	Warts may be removed by cryotherapy (freezing), podophyllin, burning, or surgery. (The viral infection remains in the body, however.)
PUBIC LICE ('crabs'): *Pthirus pubis*	Sexual contact, or by contact with an infested towel, sheet, or toilet seat	Intense itching in pubic area and other hairy regions to which lice become attached	Clinical examination	Lindane (brand name Kwell)—a prescription shampoo; nonprescription medications containing pyrethrins or piperonyl butoxide (brand names: RID, Triple X)

If left untreated, gonorrhea can spread through the genital and urinary tracts and attack the internal reproductive organs. In men, an infection of the epididymis (*epididymitis*) may occur, which sometimes can lead to infertility. The kidneys can also become involved. In women, an untreated infection can spread through the cervix to the uterus, Fallopian tubes, and, perhaps, the abdominal cavity and ovaries, which can result in *pelvic inflammatory disease* (PID).

The symptoms of PID include abdominal pain or cramps, tenderness around the abdomen or cervix, nausea, vomiting, fever, cervical discharge, irregular menstrual cycles, and pain during sexual intercourse. But some women with PID have no symptoms. With or without symptoms, PID can scar and block the Fallopian tubes, causing infertility. (Figure 3.2 on page 31 shows the relationship of the Fallopian tubes to the ovaries and the uterus). When gonorrhea is diagnosed and treated early, however, it can be cured rapidly the great majority of the time.

The first step in diagnosing gonorrhea is a medical examination. Sample discharges are then examined for bacteria. Gonorrhea is treated with, and almost always cured by, antibiotics.

Penicillin was once the favored antibiotic, but strains of gonorrhea have developed that resist penicillin. Other antibiotics are thus often used. The sex partners of people with gonorrhea should also visit the doctor and be treated, if necessary.

If you learn that you have gonorrhea or another STD, telling your partner or partners about it is the right thing to do, even if it is painful.

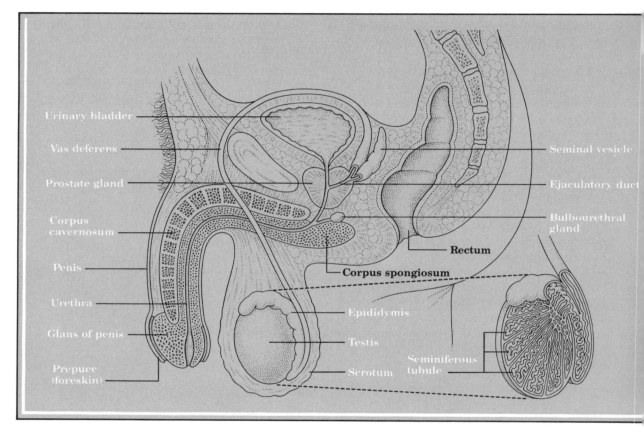

Figure 5.1. Male Sexual Anatomy. This figure provides a cross-section of the external and internal reproductive organs of the male. Sperm are produced in the seminiferous tubules. They ripen and are stored in the epididymis. Inflammation of the epididymis, which may occur in gonorrhea and other sexually transmitted diseases (STDs), can cause infertility. During ejaculation, sperm travel through the vas deferens and out of the body through the urethra. Most seminal fluid is produced by the seminal vesicles and the prostate gland. Circumcision is surgical removal of the prepuce (foreskin) of the penis. Circumcised men are apparently somewhat less likely to contract STDs.

OTHER SEXUALLY TRANSMITTED DISEASES

Syphilis

The bacterium that causes *syphilis* (pronounced SIFF-uh-liss) is *Treponema pallidum*, which derives from Greek and Latin roots meaning a 'faintly colored (pallid) turning thread.' This is a good description of the corkscrewlike pathogen as it appears under the microscope. You may hear treponema pallidum referred to as *T. pallidum* or as a 'spirochete'—another reference to its spiral shape.

The incidence of syphilis declined dramatically in the United States when penicillin was introduced, but there has been a resurgence of syphilis since the early 1980s. About 45,000 cases of syphilis are now reported each year and many others, of course, go unreported. Syphilis is much less common than gonorrhea, but its effects—when it goes untreated—can be more devastating: blindness, heart disease, mental illness, even death.

Syphilis is usually transmitted by vaginal or anal intercourse or by oral sex with an infected person. *T. pallidum* is usually transmitted through contact between the open sores of an infected person and the skin abrasions or mucous membranes of the other person's body. You can also be infected by touching an infectious *chancre*. (A chancre —pronounced SHAN-ker—is a hard, round sore with raised edges). You are not likely to catch syphilis (or gonorrhea) from a toilet seat.

Pregnant women can transmit syphilis to their babies, because *T. pallidum* can cross the placental membrane. *T. pallidum* can cause miscarriage, stillbirth, or congenital syphilis. Congenital syphilis can damage the baby's vision and hearing or deform the baby's teeth and bones. Routine blood tests during pregnancy are used to diagnose syphilis in the mother so that these problems in the baby may be averted. Babies may escape harm if their mothers are treated early in pregnancy.

Syphilis undergoes several stages of development. The first stage, or *primary stage*, is characterized by formation of a chancre at the site of infection two to four weeks after infection. In women, the chancre usually forms on the inner vaginal walls or on the cervix. But it may also appear on the external genitals, especially on the labia (see Figure 3.2, p. 29). In men, the chancre most often appears on the glans or head of the penis, but it may also develop on the shaft of the penis or on the scrotum (see Figure 5.1). If the infection is spread by oral sex, the chancre can form on the tongue or lips. If *T. pallidum* is transmitted by anal sex, a chancre can develop in the rectum. The chancre will inevitably disappear within a few weeks. If an infected person does not receive treatment, however, *T. pallidum* will continue to spread beneath the skin.

The *secondary stage* of syphilis begins within a few weeks or months and is symptomized by a rash. The rash is painless and consists of red raised bumps on the skin that darken and burst, oozing a discharge. People may also suffer from sores in the mouth, painful swelling of joints, a sore throat, headaches, and fever. Syphilis has been referred to as 'the great imitator' because these symptoms resemble a case of flu and many other illnesses.

These symptoms also disappear. Syphilis then enters a *latent stage* (latent means 'hidden') and may lie dormant for many years or a lifetime. *T. pallidum* nevertheless continues to multiply and burrow into the circulatory system, central nervous system (brain and spinal cord), and bones.

In many cases, syphilis eventually progresses to a *tertiary*, or final, stage. Large ulcers may form on various organs such as the digestive organs, liver, lungs, skin, and muscles. Yet more critical damage can occur if the infection attacks the cardiovascular system (heart and major blood vessels) or the central nervous system. Either result can be fatal. In the nervous system, syphilis can cause brain damage, resulting in paralysis or gross confusion and disorientation. The nineteenth-century French painter Paul Gauguin died from tertiary syphilis.

Because it takes time for *T. pallidum* to multiply

to large numbers, primary-stage syphilis is diagnosed by clinical examination rather than a blood test. If a chancre is found, a doctor may draw fluid from it and examine the fluid under a microscope. The spiral-shaped bacteria are usually visible.

Blood tests can diagnose syphilis when the secondary stage begins. The most frequently used blood test is the *VDRL*. As with the commonly used tests for diagnosing infection by H.I.V., the VDRL reveals the presence of antibodies to *T. pallidum* rather than the bacterium itself.

Syphilis is treated and almost always cured with penicillin or other antibiotics, even when treatment is begun in the later stages of the illness. (If you are in doubt as to whether or not you are infected, it is *not* too late to see the doctor.)

Chlamydia

Although you may have heard more about gonorrhea and syphilis, *chlamydial infections* are more common. Chlamydial infections are caused by the *Chlamydia trachomatis* bacterium, a parasitic organism that can survive only within cells. This bacterium accounts for different types of infection, including *nongonococcal urethritis* (inflammation of the urethra—abbreviated NGU) in women and men; *cervicitis* (inflammation of the cervix), *endometritis* (inflammation of the endometrium), and PID in women; and epididymitis in men.

It is estimated that there may be as many as 4 million cases of chlamydial infections each year in the United States. The incidence of chlamydial infections among teenagers and college students is especially high.

Chlamydial infections are usually transmitted sexually through vaginal or anal intercourse. *Chlamydia trachomatis* can also infect the eyes if a person touches her or his eyes after touching the genitals of an infected partner. Chlamydia can also invade the throat, so couples are advised not to engage in oral sex if one of the partners is infected with chlamydia. Babies can acquire chlamydial eye infections as they pass through the cervix of an infected mother during childbirth.

The symptoms of chlamydial infections closely resemble those of gonorrhea, although they are usually milder. Although *Chlamydia trachomatis* can inflame the urethras of both women and men, the infection is usually referred to as nongonococcal urethritis in men only. Women are usually said to have a chlamydial infection or simply chlamydia. *Urethritis* is an inflammation of the urethra, which is the canal through which urine passes from the bladder to the outside world. Nongonococcal urethritis or NGU refers to any type of urethritis that is *not* caused by the gonococcal bacterium. Many organisms can cause NGU, but *Chlamydia trachomatis* is the most common.

Men with NGU may notice a thin, whitish discharge (as contrasted to the yellow-green gonococcal discharge) from the penis and some pain or burning sensations during urination (not as intense as with gonorrhea, however). They may have feelings of heaviness in the testes and soreness in the scrotum.

In women, chlamydial infections generally involve infections of the urethra (*urethritis*) or cervix (*cervicitis*). Women may experience burning urination, a mild vaginal discharge, pelvic pain, irritation in the genitals, and disruption of the menstrual cycle. The cervix may appear swollen and inflamed to a doctor. Oral sex with an infected partner may cause a sore throat in either sex.

Although such symptoms are possible, only about one in three women and men who are infected with chlamydia actually have them. Because so many people are symptom-free, chlamydia has been dubbed the 'silent disease.' People with chlamydial infections can unwittingly transmit them to their sex partners, who in turn may unknowingly infect others.

When untreated, chlamydia can spread to the woman's internal reproductive organs, causing PID, which, in turn, can cause infertility because of obstructing the Fallopian tubes. Perhaps half of the 1.25 million cases of PID diagnosed each year are caused by chlamydial infections. Untreated gonorrhea is also a major cause.

In men, untreated chlamydial infections can also damage reproductive organs, such as the epididymis. About half of the cases of epididymitis can be traced to chlamydial infections. Epididymitis may be characterized by swelling, feelings of tenderness, pain in the scrotum, and fever.

Diagnosis and treatment are summarized in Table 5.1.

VAGINITIS

Vaginitis refers to any kind of vaginal infection or inflammation. Vaginitis is usually known by the presence of a foul-smelling discharge. Other symptoms may include genital itching or irritation, and burning during urination.

Some cases of vaginitis are caused by allergic reactions or sensitivities to chemicals. Most, however, are caused by infectious agents that are transmitted sexually or naturally reside in the vagina but 'overgrow' when the normal environmental balance of the vagina is upset. The use of antibiotics or birth-control pills, changes in diet, excessive douching, or pantyhose or nylon underwear can produce vaginal changes that allow infectious microorganisms to multiply.

The majority of vaginal infections involve bacterial vaginosis, candidiasis (yeast infections), trichomoniasis, or some combination of the three.

Preventing a Vaginal Infection

Women readers with vaginitis are advised to consult their gynecologists. Nevertheless, the following suggestions may help prevent vaginitis:

1. Wash your external genitals regularly with mild soap.

2. Wear cotton panties (nylon underwear retains heat and moisture that allow organisms that produce vaginitis to grow).

3. Avoid clothes that are tight in the crotch.

4. If you are sexually active, be certain that your sex partner is well washed. Condoms can help reduce the probability of being infected by one's sex partner.

5. Use K-Y jelly or another sterile, water-soluble if artificial lubrication is needed for sexual activity. Avoid Vaseline. (Birth-control jellies are also appropriate as lubricants.)

6. Discontinue sexual activity that feels painful or abrasive.

7. Avoid diets that are high in sugar and refined carbohydrates. They can alter the normal pH of the vagina and permit organisms that cause vaginal infections to overgrow.

8. Women who are subject to vaginal infections may find it beneficial to douche from time to time with plain water, a solution of baking soda, or of a tablespoon or two of vinegar in about a quart of warm water. Douches of unpasteurized, unflavored yogurt can help resupply the 'good' bacteria that are normally located in the vagina but that may have been killed off by antibiotics. Do not douche if you are pregnant or suspect that you might be. Check with your gynecologist before douching.

9. Pay attention to your general health. Poor diet and lack of sleep can lower your resistance to infection.

Bacterial Vaginosis

Bacterial vaginosis (referred to as *nonspecific vaginitis* until quite recently) is most often caused by the *Gardnerella vaginalis* bacterium. This bacterium is usually transmitted sexually. In women, it often gives rise to a thin, odorous vaginal discharge, but the disease can also be asymptomatic. Diagnosis relies on culturing the bacterium in the laboratory. Physicians usually recommend oral treatment for seven days with metronidazole (brand name Flagyl). Treatment is usually effective, but recurrences are common.

Candidiasis

Candidiasis—also known as *moniliasis, thrush,* or a yeast infection—is caused by the yeast-like fungus, *Candida albicans*. Candidiasis commonly produces symptoms of inflammation, soreness, and intense itching in the genital area. There is also a white, curd-like vaginal discharge. Although fungus is almost always present to some degree, it generally causes no problems or symptoms when the vaginal environment is normal.

Symptoms most often arise when changes in the vaginal environment permit the fungus to overgrow. Pregnancy, diabetes, and the use of birth-control pills or antibiotics often change the chemical balance of the vagina. Nylon underwear and restrictive, poorly ventilated clothing may also encourage yeast infections.

Candidiasis can be transmitted sexually and bounced back and forth between sex partners. Sex partners should thus be treated simultaneously. Candidiasis in men usually takes the form of NGU, of reddening of the penis, or of genital thrush such that it burns and itches to urinate. Candidiasis can also be transmitted nonsexually, as when women share a damp washcloth. Candidiasis can also be transmitted back and forth between the genitals and the mouth through oral sex, and to the anus through anal sex.

Diet apparently plays a role. Eating less of substances that produce large amounts of urinary sugar (less sugar, dairy products, and artificial sweeteners, for example) seems to reduce the recurrence of yeast infections.

Candidiasis is very common. As many as three college women in four will have at least one occurrence of candidiasis. Perhaps half will have recurrent infections. Gynecologists usually recommend three days of treatment with vaginal suppositories, tablets, or creams containing miconazole (brand name Monistat), clotrimazole (brand names Lotrimin and Mycelex), or teraconazole (brand name Terazol).

Trichomoniasis

Trichomoniasis, or 'trich,' is a vaginal infection caused by a parasite—a protozoan (one-celled animal) called *Trichomonas vaginalis*. There are about 8 million cases of trichomoniasis each year among American women. Symptoms include itching or burning sensations in the genital region, and a foamy whitish to yellow-green discharge that is often foul-smelling. Mild pain may occur during intercourse or urination. About 50 percent of infected women report no symptoms, however.

Trichomoniasis is almost always transmitted sexually. It can cause NGU in men, either producing no symptoms or a slight penile discharge which is generally noticeable only in the morning before first urination. There may also be slight irritation of the urethra and sensations of itching or tingling in the urethral tract. Since men may carry 'trich' without realizing it, they are capable of unknowingly infecting their sex partners. It is also possible to pick up trich from contact with infected semen on washcloths, towels, or bedclothes. It is remotely possible to pick up trich from a toilet seat, but the organism would have to come into direct contact with the penis or woman's genital organs. Diagnosis can be made in the doctor's office on the basis of microscopic examination of a smear of the woman's vaginal secretions. The examination of cultures grown from the sample is considered the most sensitive method of diagnosis.

Trichomoniasis is treated in women and men with metronidazole (brand name Flagyl), except during the first trimester of pregnancy.

Because couples may bounce the infection back and forth, both should be treated, whether or not they report symptoms. Treatment is considered nearly 100 percent effective if both sex partners are treated.

STDs Caused by Viruses

AIDS is caused by the human immunodeficiency virus (H.I.V.). Many other kinds of viruses also give rise to STDs. Let us consider herpes, viral hepatitis, and genital warts.

Herpes

The *Herpes simplex* virus causes different kinds of herpes. The most common kind, *Herpes simplex virus type 1* (H.S.V.-1 virus), causes oral herpes, which gives rise to cold sores or fever blisters in the mouth or on the lips. H.S.V.-1 can be transmitted to the genitals by touch or oral sex.

Genital herpes is caused by a related virus— *Herpes simplex virus type 2* (H.S.V.-2). H.S.V.-2 produces painful blisters and sores on the genitals. H.S.V.-2 can also be transmitted to the mouth by means of oral sex.

More than 100 million Americans have been infected with H.S.V.-1. Ten to twenty million have been infected with H.S.V.-2. There may be half a million new case of genital herpes in the United States each year. Although you might assume that better-educated people are less likely to contract STDs, genital herpes is actually more common among people who are better-educated, such as college students. Many students are thus concerned about herpes and its potential effects on future relationships.

Herpes can be transmitted by means of vaginal, oral, or anal sex, or by touching herpes sores. Touching a sore and then touching one's eyes can cause a potentially serious eye infection. Herpes viruses also survive for many hours on objects such as toilet seats, and they can be spread by contact with these objects. Oral herpes may be transmitted by kissing, by sharing a drinking cup as an infected person, or by sharing a towel. Genital herpes is usually transmitted sexually, however.

Flare-ups of genital herpes can come and go, giving rise to genital sores and to feelings of itching and burning. People are more contagious during such outbreaks. But genital herpes may also be sexually transmitted even in the absence of symptoms.

Since H.S.V.-2 cannot pass through a latex condom, sexually active couples are advised to use condoms during flare-ups. Spermicides with nonoxynol-9 also kill H.S.V.; condoms combined with this spermicide thus provide double protection. Condoms do not protect men when their scrotums touch sores or infected vaginal secretions, however.

Women with herpes infections are about three times more likely than uninfected women to have miscarriages. Babies may also be infected with genital herpes during childbirth—an infection that can be fatal to a newborn baby. Obstetricians usually recommend Caesarean sections to protect the baby if the mother has a flare-up of genital herpes at time of delivery. The Caesarean allows the baby to avoid the infected birth canal (vagina). Herpes also apparently places women at greater risk for cancers of the genital organs, such as cancer of the cervix.

Symptoms appear about six to eight days after infection in the form of genital sores. The sores are at first painful red bumps on the vulva or the penis. Sores may also be found on the buttocks or thigh, in the vagina, or on the cervix. These sores become groups of small fluid-filled blisters. The fluid contains infectious viral particles. When the blisters are attacked by the immune system, they fill with pus and break open. At this time they become shallow, painful sores that are surrounded with a red ring. People are especially infectious during this stage, because the sores shed millions of viral particles. H.S.V.-2 can also cause headaches, muscle aches, fever, swollen lymph glands, burning urination, and a vaginal discharge. Herpes blisters normally crust over and heal within a few weeks.

Although the symptoms disappear, H.S.V.-2 does not. H.S.V.-2 burrows into nerve cells in the spine, where it can lie dormant for many years. Infected people are considered least contagious when the disease is dormant.

One piece of good news is that about half of the people who are infected with H.S.V.-2 have only one flare-up of genital herpes. When recurrences occur, they usually do so within a year and affect the same area of the body. Recurrences are usually briefer and milder than the initial outbreak. Although recurrences tend to become less common over the years, some people have frequent flare-ups.

Doctors initially diagnose genital herpes by examining the sores or ulcers that appear during an outbreak. They may also take a sample of fluid from a sore for further examination.

We have no cure or vaccine for herpes. Viruses do not respond to antibiotics. There are a number of antiviral drugs, however. One of them— acyclovir (brand name Zovirax)—helps relieve discomfort and fosters healing. Acyclovir can be applied directly to the sores to reduce the duration of viral shedding (the amount of time during H.S.V.-2 is found in semen and in vaginal secretions). Acyclovir can also be taken in pill form to combat internal sores in the vagina and on the cervix. Acyclovir tablets can reduce the inten-

sity of the first episode and the frequency and duration of subsequent outbreaks.

Other measures such as warm baths, loose fitting clothing, and wet compresses may help relieve discomfort during flare-ups.

The emotional consequences of genital herpes can be more disturbing than the physical symptoms. Many sufferers, for example, worry about a lifetime of outbreaks and whether they will be able to marry a person who is not also infected with genital herpes.

In one anonymous survey, more than half of the Brooklyn College students who identified themselves as having genital herpes reported strong emotional reactions to the disease.[3] Most reported strong feelings of anger and fear. Half reported that they felt damaged. Three in four reported that herpes had led them to avoid sex for a long time, but most became sexually active again. The majority of herpes sufferers reported seeking partners who also had herpes so that they would not risk transmitting the disease to uninfected persons.

Some herpes sufferers are helped by support groups that share ways of living with the disease. A caring and trusting partner is also important.

Viral Hepatitis

There are a number of kinds of *hepatitis* (inflammations of the liver). They are caused by different viruses and are often sexually transmitted. The major kinds are *hepatitis A, B, C,* and *D.*

Hepatitis A infections are usually temporary and characterized by jaundice (a condition in which the skin, urine, and eyeballs take on a yellow hue because of abnormally high amounts of bile pigments in the blood), abdominal discomfort, weakness and nausea, loss of appetite, and whitish bowel movements. Hepatitis B is more severe and enduring. Hepatitis C involves milder symptoms. People with hepatitis C may not have jaundice, but they may incur chronic liver disease or cancer of the liver. Hepatitis D occurs only along with hepatitis B. The symptoms are similar to those of hepatitis B but may be more life-threatening.

Hepatitis A and B can be transmitted sexually, primarily through sexual activity that involves the anus. Hepatitis A is transmitted mainly through contact with infected fecal matter (bowel movements), as found in contaminated food or water. Sexual transmission of hepatitis A usually involves oral–anal sex (licking the anal opening). Sexual transmission of hepatitis B usually involves oral–anal sex and anal intercourse (insertion of the penis into the anus). Hepatitis B may also be transmitted by means of transfusion with contaminated blood, sharing contaminated needles (as among people who shoot up drugs), and by semen, saliva, menstrual blood, and nasal mucus. Hepatitis C can also be transmitted sexually. Hepatitis D can be transmitted through sexual activity or contact with infected blood.

Hepatitis is usually diagnosed by means of blood tests that screen for abnormalities in liver functioning. There is no cure for viral hepatitis, but bed rest and fluids are usually recommended. A vaccine provides protection against hepatitis B and also against hepatitis D, because hepatitis D cannot occur in the absence of hepatitis B. There is no vaccine for hepatitis C.

Genital Warts

Genital warts (also called *venereal warts*) are caused by the human papilloma virus (H.P.V.). It is estimated that 20 to 30 percent of sexually active people in the United States are infected with H.P.V.[4] Genital warts are found most often in women and men aged 20 to 24. They appear around the genitals and anus within a few months of infection. Women are more vulnerable to infection than men because an area of cells in the cervix undergoes relatively rapid cell division, and H.P.V. uses dividing cells to reproduce itself.

Women who begin to have sexual intercourse before the age of 18 and who have multiple sex partners are especially vulnerable to H.P.V. A recent study of women visiting the health center at the University of California at Berkeley found that 46 percent of them were infected with H.P.V.[5] In some cities, about half (yes, *half*) of the sexually active teenage girls appear to be infected.

Genital warts are similar to the common plantar warts and consist of itchy bumps of various shapes and sizes. The warts tend be hard and yellow-gray on areas of dry skin, and soft, pinkish and cauliflower-shaped in moist areas, as in the vagina. They can be found on the penis, foreskin, scrotum, and inside the urethra of men. In women they may be found on the labia majora and minora, the vaginal wall, and the cervix. Men and women may also find them outside the genital region—on the lips, in the mouth, on the eyelids, on the nipples, around the anus, or in the rectum.

Genital warts that form on the urethra can cause painful discharges or bleeding. H.P.V. may also give rise to cancer in the genital tract, as in the cases of cancers of the penis or cervix.

H.P.V. can be transmitted through sexual and other kinds of contact, as through contact with infected clothing or towels. Genital warts are often removed by means of freezing (*cryotherapy*) with liquid nitrogen. The warts can also be repeatedly dabbed with a podophyllin solution to make them dry up and fall off. Physicians may also burn warts off with electrodes or remove them surgically—either by knife or laser beam. These treatments remove the warts, but they do not eradicate H.P.V. from the body. Genital warts may thus recur.

H.P.V. has been linked to cancer of the cervix. It is found in the majority of women who develop cervical cancer. Health professionals advise women to protect themselves from H.P.V.-related cervical cancer by having regular Pap smears for early detection and by limiting their number of sex partners.

STDs Caused by Parasites

Parasites are larger than the bacteria, viruses, protozoa, and fungi that cause other STDs. They can become troublesome because the body generally lacks natural forms of defense against them. It is thus nearly impossible to get rid of them without medical treatment.

Fortunately, drugs are available that kill most parasites, including ones that are transmitted sexually. It is important for you to know about the common parasitic infestation caused by pubic lice.

Pubic Lice

Pubic lice have been dubbed 'crabs' because of their appearance under a microscope. (You can also see them with the naked eye.)

Pubic lice belong to a family of insects called biting lice that also includes head lice and body lice. Head lice cling to the hair of the scalp and are often spread among schoolchildren. Pubic lice are often spread sexually, but they may also be transmitted by coming into contact with infested towels, sheets, or—yes—toilet seats. Pubic lice can survive for only a day or so without a human host.

They lay eggs that can take a week to hatch in bedding or towels, however. All bedding, clothes, and towels that have been used by an infested person should therefore be washed in hot water or dry-cleaned to kill and remove eggs.

'Crabs' attach themselves to pubic hair and feed on the blood of their hosts, often causing itching. Their life span is short, only a month or so. They are prolific breeders, however, and may lay eggs many times before they die.

Pubic lice may be treated with a prescription medication (brand name Kwell), which comes in a cream, lotion, or shampoo. They may also be eradicated with nonprescription preparations that contain pyrethrins or piperonyl butoxide. Brand names include RID, NIX, and Triple X.

Now that you have learned about AIDS, other STDs, and the organisms that give rise to them, perhaps you will agree that the wisest way to cope with them is to avoid infection in the first place. Avoiding infection is what is meant by *prevention*. Prevention is the subject of Chapter 6.

6 Prevention

Since there are no vaccines and no cures for H.I.V. infection and AIDS, the best approach to dealing with them is prevention. Prevention has focused on three major avenues of transmission: (1) sexual contact, (2) injection ('shooting up') of drugs, and (3) blood transfusions. The effort to make blood supplies safe through testing potential donors has nearly eliminated the threat of infection from blood transfusions. Efforts to reduce the risk of infection through sexual relations and injection of drugs have had mixed results.

AIDS has forced us to confront our sexual behavior and take responsibility for our sexual interactions as never before. Prevention efforts have largely focused on educating people about H.I.V. and AIDS and encouraging sexually active people to limit their numbers of partners and use safer sex techniques, such as 'outercourse' and intercourse with latex condoms.

The extent of unprotected sex on college campuses remains unknown. Evidence suggests, however, that the threat of AIDS has not greatly affected the sexual behavior of most college students:

- Fewer than half of a sample of University of Rhode Island students reported changing their sexual behavior because of the threat of AIDS.[1] The most commonly reported change was becoming more selective in choice of partners.
- Surveys of college women treated at a student health service in a northeastern university in 1975, 1986, and 1989 also showed little change in such sexual practices as engaging in sexual relations with multiple partners.[2] The majority of sexually active women seen at this clinic also did not use condoms regularly.
- A survey at the University of Massachusetts found that nearly seven of ten students reported that they had *not* changed their sexual practices because of AIDS.[3]
- A survey of students at two southeastern state universities found that only 35 percent of sexually active students used condoms regularly.[4]
- A large-scale survey of over 5,500 first-year college students in fifty-one postsecondary institutions in Canada reported

that only 24.8 percent of the men and 15.6 percent of the women always used a condom when they engaged in sexual relations.[5] One in five men and one in eleven women reported having ten or more sex partners. Among this sub-group, only one in five men and fewer than one in ten women regularly used condoms. Despite their behavior, the students were generally knowledgeable about transmission of H.I.V.

Why do so many sexually active young people fail to protect themselves from H.I.V. infection? Perhaps the threat of AIDS flies out of their minds when there is an opportunity for sex. Perhaps they assume that they and their partners are not infected. Perhaps a condom isn't handy. Perhaps they feel that a condom is too much trouble, or they are too embarrassed to buy one. Perhaps the men do not want to decrease their sexual sensations. Perhaps they assume that they are too young and vibrant to contract AIDS.

The adventurous spirit that we connect with youth may confer a sense of immortality and a greater willingness to take risks.

Former Surgeon General C. Everett Koop advised that the two certain paths to avoiding sexual transmission of H.I.V. are celibacy (or abstinence) and maintaining a lifelong monogamous relationship with an uninfected person. In this chapter we talk about abstinence and monogamy. We also discuss safer sex and resisting sexual pressure.

First, our students often ask us what is meant by abstinence. Abstinence from what? We'll see that there is no easy answer. Even the issue of monogamy is more complex than it might at first appear. After all, many readers still have to get to there (monogamy, that is) from here—from being a virgin (or a 'technical virgin,' that is). What is 'safe sex,' and just how safe is it? Are abstinence, monogamy, and safe sex 'certain paths' to avoiding infection with H.I.V.? What is sexual pressure, and why do we talk about it in a book on STDs? You will see why.

ABSTINENCE—WHAT IS IT?

We looked up 'abstinence' in the dictionary. It was defined as voluntarily doing without *some* or *all* food, drink, or 'other pleasures.' In an article on safer sex, *Newsweek* magazine defined abstinence more simply—'Don't do it,' the magazine said.[6]

'Don't do it'? Don't do *what*? Don't hold hands? Don't kiss? Don't tongue kiss? Don't pet above the waist? Below the waist? Our students have asked us, 'Just what does abstinence mean?' There is also a related question: What are the risks connected with the different meanings of abstinence?

Return to the dictionary. Abstinence can mean doing without *some* or *all* of certain kinds of pleasures, including the pleasures of romance and sex. We can assume that abstinence is a 'certain

path' to avoiding infection with H.I.V. when couples abstain from all sexual activity other than holding hands—so long as a hand is not bleeding and so long as the infected blood does not find its way into the bloodstream of one's partner through sores or cracks in the skin, the mouth, or other parts of the body. These are very remote possibilities, of course, but we mention them just to remind readers that no two situations are exactly alike, and that they need to maintain an awareness of how H.I.V. is transmitted.

In the section on 'outercourse' that comes later, we'll talk about hugging, kissing, and petting—all of which are used by many students who consider themselves to be abstaining from sex—sexual intercourse, that is.

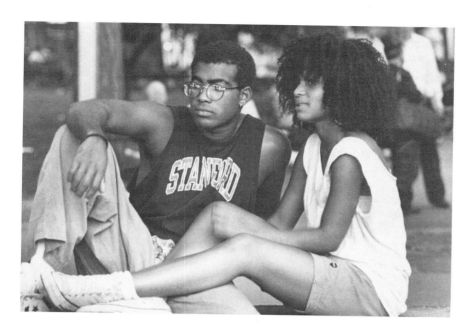

Choices—Abstinence? A Lifelong Monogamous Relationship? Safe(r) Sex? Given that there is no cure or effective vaccine for AIDS, prevention is clearly the wisest course. But prevention has many meanings, and college students need to decide whether, and how, they will attempt to prevent AIDS and other sexually transmitted diseases.

A LIFELONG MONOGAMOUS RELATIONSHIP —HOW DO YOU GET THERE FROM HERE?

If you limit sexual activity to a lifelong monogamous relationship with a person who is not infected with H.I.V., you will be safe enough from sexual transmission of H.I.V. The big questions are: What have you done already? And, if you have never engaged in sexual relations with anyone, how do you get from where you are today to that 'lifelong monogamous relationship' with a person who is not infected with H.I.V.?

Once upon a time, sex (at least for women) was limited to marriage just like rapid transportation was limited to the horse and carriage. Surveys of the sexual behavior of young people do not all agree in their findings. It seems safe to conclude, however, that the majority of young people of both sexes today engage in sexual relations before they get married. Girls and young women are more likely than boys and young men to limit sexual relations to people they care about or intend to marry. Nevertheless, even if you are a virgin when you get married, it does not mean that your partner will be. Even if you and your partner both marry as virgins—or at least without ever having had sexual relations with anyone else—one of you may have one or more extramarital affairs.

Some readers will also be what was once called 'technical virgins' when they get married. They may never have engaged in sexual intercourse, but they may have engaged in deep kissing and forms of heavy petting that carry some risk of transmitting H.I.V.

If you think we are saying that there is no such thing as a lifelong monogamous relationship with an uninfected partner, that is wrong. Such relationships are possible, but they may be rarer than you think. Also keep in mind that we are promoting saf*er* sex, not perfectly safe sex, because perfectly safe sex, like other perfectionistic ideals, may be beyond the grasp of most readers. Our message is this: You are less likely to be infected with H.I.V. if you have one sex partner rather than many sex partners—especially if your partner also has limited sexual experience.

When in doubt, you and your intended lifelong partner can be tested for infection with H.I.V. —more than once, if necessary.

THE TRUTH ABOUT 'SAFE SEX'—IT'S REALLY SAF*ER* SEX

There are many ways of reducing the risk of sexual transmission of H.I.V. None of these suggestions can be certified as rendering sexual contact perfectly safe, however. Despite the commonly heard buzz words 'safe sex,' we can speak only of saf*er* sex—not of foolproof safe sex. There are no guarantees.

Be Discerning in Your Choice of Sex Partners

Be discriminating in your sex partners. Avoid sexual contact with people who are known to be infected with H.I.V. Avoid sexual contact with people whom are known to have done things—or whom you suspect of having done things—that place them at risk of being infected. If you have no idea about your partner's history, you may not know enough about her or him to be safe.

Uninfected people are not at risk of transmitting the infection, regardless of their histories. The problem is that you may not know, and probably do not know for certain, whether a person is free of H.I.V. Finding out—learning whether someone has engaged in risky behavior may require the kind of intimate knowledge that takes a good deal of time to develops. It is probably not enough to ask a potential sex partner about her or his past sexual behavior and use of drugs, for example. You need to know her or him well enough to assess the truthfulness of her or his answers. Even then, you cannot be absolutely certain that you are being told the truth. It is even possible that the potential partner does not know everything about her or his own past. It is conceivable, for example, that she or he might have received a contaminated blood transfusion after an auto accident several years back. To be perfectly safe, it is necessary to abstain from sex with a partner who is not absolutely known to be uninfected. To be 'mostly safe,' one must at least practice safer sex techniques with a partner until it becomes evident that the possibility of being infected with H.I.V. is extremely remote.

One way to make the possibility of being infected extremely remote is for you and your partner to be tested for H.I.V. antibodies before you initiate a sexual relationship. But then you have to keep in mind the fact that blood tests for H.I.V. antibodies may not yield positive results for several months after a person has been infected. It may thus make sense to observe caution even after a single negative test result.

Does it sound as if we're placing impossible hurdles in your path? Does it just seem like too much to ask someone you care about to take a blood test now and then take another test in half a year or so before you initiate sexual relations? In the United States of the 1990s, it may indeed be asking much. But what is 'too much' when your life and the lives of your children may depend on it? Moreover, you can engage in protected sex until repeated test results are negative.

Avoid Sexual Activity with Multiple Partners

No mystery here. The greater the number of sexual contacts, the more likely it is that one or more will be with someone who is infected. Then, too, how can you be discerning about your choice of multiple partners? It is similarly advisable to avoid sex with someone who has had multiple partners.

How, you may wonder, can you know whether your partner has had (or currently has) multiple partners? Again, it may not be enough just to ask. As noted in Chapter 4, many people admit that they would lie about their sexual histories in order to convince someone to engage in sexual activity. Here, too, the answer is to take some time before becoming sexually involved. As the relationship deepens, you will find many clues as to your partner's history—sexual and otherwise. You will

also develop a sense of whether things are being withheld from you. As you get to know that person's friends and acquaintances, they may also provide useful pieces of information, even without being asked to do so. (In George Bernard Shaw's play, *Caesar and Cleopatra*, a character asks Julius Caesar whether a prisoner should be tortured to make him reveal needed information. The problem, responds Caesar, is not making people reveal information—it is getting them to be silent! The tendency to reveal information is also found within circles of friends and acquaintances.)

In short, you are likely to learn a great deal about a prospective sex partner as time goes on. The question is whether you are willing to wait for such information and then believe it, or whether you are so attracted, and so afraid of losing her or him, that you rush into something that you might regret. (If you read between the lines here, you'll realize that we're talking about a great deal more than sexually transmitted diseases.)

Use 'Protection'

Just what is *protected* sex? The term *protected* is used in different ways, but almost everyone will agree that protected sexual intercourse at the very least means intercourse with the use of a latex condom. Some people say that protected sex should include a condom in combination with a spermicide that contains nonoxynol-9 or octoxynol, because these are toxic to H.I.V. (They kill H.I.V. as well as sperm.)

Remember that 'protection' is advisable not only for intercourse in which the penis is placed in the vagina. Unprotected oral-genital activity (oral sex) and oral-anal activity are also considered to place people at high risk of being infected with H.I.V.

A number of devices that are basically intended to prevent unwanted pregnancies also provide some protection against transmission of H.I.V. through sexual intercourse. These include male and female condoms and, to some extent, the diaphragm in combination with a spermicide. Spermicides alone are probably better than no protection at all, but they should be used in combination with condoms.

Male condoms are also called 'rubbers,' 'safes,' 'prophylactics' (because latex condoms protect against STDs), and 'skins' (referring to condoms that are made from animal membranes). Latex condoms can help prevent the spread of AIDS and other STDs by serving as a barrier to the disease-causing microorganisms, including H.I.V. Although latex condoms can be said to afford 'good' protection against transmission of H.I.V. and other disease-causing organisms, they are not considered 100 percent effective in preventing the transmission of H.I.V. This is one of the reasons that we speak of 'safer sex' and not of perfectly safe sex.

Condoms are easy to get (no prescription needed) from pharmacies and family-planning clinics—even from vending machines that are found in some college dormitories. Some AIDS-prevention programs and school districts distribute free condoms in the belief that easier access to condoms will encourage their use and thus reduce the risk of H.I.V. transmission. New York City makes condoms available to high-school students, with or without parental knowledge or permission. The Los Angeles school district provides condoms for high-school students with parental permission.

Some condoms are made of latex rubber. Thinner, more expensive condoms ('skins') are made from the intestinal membranes of animals. Condoms that are made from animal membranes allow greater sexual sensations (sex feels more exciting or 'natural' with them). They do not protect you as well from STDs, however. Only latex condoms form an effective barrier to H.I.V. (Condoms made of animal intestines may have pores large enough to permit H.I.V. and other pathogens to slip through.) Some condoms are plain-tipped, and others have nipples or reservoirs that catch semen and may help prevent the condom from bursting during ejaculation.

The condom is a sheath that serves as a barrier, preventing the passage of disease-carrying micro-organisms (and sperm) from the man to his partner. They also help prevent infected vaginal fluids

(and microorganisms) from entering the man's urethral opening (the hole in the tip of the penis; see Figure 5.1) or from penetrating through small cracks in the skin of the penis.

The condom is rolled onto the penis once erection is achieved and before contact occurs between the penis and the vagina. Don't engage in sexual intercourse until just before ejaculation and fool yourself into thinking that either of you is protected! Before ejaculation, some semen may already have passed into the vagina. Vaginal fluids have already come into contact with the penis. The condom is used most effectively when the couple:

- Unroll the condom onto the erect penis before the penis touches one's sex partner.
- Leave a half inch of space at the tip of a plain-ended condom where the semen can accumulate.
- Use only water-based lubricants like K-Y jelly (oil-based lubricants can decrease the elasticity of latex condoms, causing them to tear).
- Carefully withdraw the penis from the vagina while it is still erect, shortly after ejaculation.
- Hold the rim of the condom when the penis is withdrawn to prevent the condom from slipping (and allowing semen to escape into the vagina).
- Check for tears in the condom before throwing it away. If the condom falls or slips off, or if any tears are found, a spermicide (which also kills H.I.V. and many other pathogens) should be used right away. (Keep some handy.)

Condoms have many advantages. They are available as needed. They can be bought without prescription. They require no special fitting and can remain in sealed packages until needed. They are easily discarded after they are used. The combination of condoms and spermicides containing nonoxynol-9 or octoxynol greatly increases protection against STD-causing organisms, including H.I.V. When in doubt, ask the pharmacist.

People do have some complaints about condoms. For one thing, condoms may make sex less spontaneous. When you're all ready to engage in intercourse, you have to stop to put it on. Moreover, if you're not sure of yourself, putting the condom on carefully is just one more thing that you can 'mess up.' You should know, however, that some couples enjoy sharing fitting the condom. They find it an erotic aspect of making love.

Condoms also lessen sexual sensations somewhat, especially for the man. That is why the thinner condoms made of animal membrane are preferred by many men. The great majority of young men, however, still obtain enough sexual stimulation to find intercourse very enjoyable. When you consider everything to be gained from wearing a condom, the loss of *some* sexual sensation is not very significant at all.

Inspect Your Partner's Sex Organs

There are unlikely to be any local telltale signs of infection with H.I.V. Nevertheless, people who are infected with H.I.V. are also often infected with organisms that cause other STDs, and these STDs often do have telltale signs. Check your partner's sex organs for rashes, chancres, blisters, discharges, warts, and lice during foreplay. Consider any disagreeable odor a warning sign. At the very least, an obnoxious odor may mean that your partner is not very clean. An unpleasant odor can also be a sign of several kinds of STDs, however.

Isn't it difficult to inspect your partner's genitals in the back seat of a car, you may ask, or under similar unwieldy circumstances? True enough. We can only answer your question with another question. Could it be that the need to engage in sexual relations under rushed or inconvenient circumstances may be in itself a warning sign? If you cannot make sex comfortable and reasonably safe, is it possible that you are not ready for sex?

Engage in 'Outercourse,' not 'Intercourse'

You know what intercourse is, so what is 'outercourse'? *Outercourse* is a term that was just recently coined and refers to any kind of sexual activity in which nothing is inserted into a person. More specifically, in outercourse no tongue, finger, or penis is inserted into any mouth, vagina, or anus.

Forms of outercourse include massage, hugging, caressing, mutual masturbation (either masturbating in one another's presence or massaging one's partner to orgasm), and rubbing bodies together without vaginal, anal, or oral contact. These are all relatively low-risk ways of finding sexual pleasure. Sharing sexual fantasies and intimate talk can be highly erotic. So can showering or bathing together—as long as semen or vaginal fluids touch only healthy skin. Even tiny cuts can allow penetration by H.I.V. and other STD-causing organisms.

Hugging with clothing on can be considered a safe way of obtaining some pleasure because there is no documented case of a person being infected in this way. Hugging in the nude may also be considered safe in itself, although nude hugging has a way of leading to other things.

Most forms of light and heavy petting are also likely to be safe enough—at least the great majority of the time. Kissing—which may be considered a form of light petting—is unlikely to transmit H.I.V., although the risk is greater when you place your tongues in each others' mouths or share large amounts of saliva.

Touching, rubbing, or stroking your partner's breasts or sex organs is not likely to transmit H.I.V., but some ways of petting are clearly more risky than others. For example, kissing, licking, or sucking the breasts could theoretically allow infected saliva to enter a woman's body through the pores (tiny openings) in the areola—the dark area that circles the nipple. Biting the breasts, as in 'love bites,' may create small wounds and increase the possibility of infection. Inserting fingers into the vagina can infect either partner if there are tiny cuts or scrapes in the fingers. (Infected blood from the fingers could enter the vagina; infected vaginal fluids could enter the partner's bloodstream through the cuts in the fingers.) Rough fingering of the vagina can also easily cut or scrape the vaginal walls, increasing the risk of infection with H.I.V. and other microorganisms.

There are also some cases in which kissing, licking, or sucking the penis or the woman's sex organs (the vagina, the major and minor lips, and the other structures surrounding the vagina) have apparently transmitted H.I.V.

Heavy petting may be risky when the man ejaculates on the skin of his partner, as in his partner's hand or against her (or his) body. Infected semen could find its way into his partner's bloodstream through cuts and scrapes on the skin. If you're going to do this, you may want to gently wash or wipe off the semen with a tissue, a towel, or a stream of running water. Don't use a tissue or something else and rub the semen off violently—you could abrade your skin in the process.

Use Barrier Devices When You Engage in Oral Sex

If you are going to practice oral sex, use a barrier device to prevent transmission of H.I.V. Apply a male latex condom before kissing, licking, or sucking a penis. Use what is referred to as a dental dam (ask the pharmacist) before kissing, licking,

or sucking the vagina or the structures surrounding the vagina. If you cannot get hold of a dental dam, a thin plastic sheet such as Saran Wrap is better than nothing, but we cannot recommend it as desirable or sufficient.

Avoid Sex When You Are in Doubt

None of the 'safer sex' measures we have listed guarantees protection from H.I.V. and other disease-causing organisms. We generally recommend that you avoid any sexual activity about which you are in doubt. Being in doubt may mean that you are in doubt about your partner. Why engage in sexual activity with someone you don't know very well, or with someone you have mixed feelings about?

Why don't you wait a while and try to sort out your feelings? Or try to get answers to questions you might have about your potential sex partner? Being in doubt may also mean that you are unsure about how safe the sexual activity is. You can always refresh your memory by referring to these pages now and then. You can also limit sexual activity to some highly safe forms of outercourse until you have had a chance to think things through. You can engage in shallow kissing, for example, coupled, perhaps, with petting through your clothing. Ironically, petting with your clothing on is safer than kissing, although it may seem like you're getting the horse before the cart. When in doubt about all this, why not express your concerns to your partner. *If you feel that your partner will not be receptive to talking about these things with you, that's an excellent reason for thinking about finding another partner!*

RESISTING SEXUAL PRESSURE: WHAT IT IS, WHAT TO DO

What do you do if your date doesn't seem to want to take no for an answer? What do you do if your date says, 'If you don't have sex, I'll find someone who will'?

We have discussed the roles of abstinence, monogamy, and safer sex in preventing the transmission of H.I.V. All of that information can fly out the window, unfortunately, if you are coerced or pressured into sexual activity.

Knowing what H.I.V. does to the body and how it is transmitted may not be enough. Abstinence, monogamy, and safer sex may not be enough. You also have to be aware of the types of sexual pressure you may encounter, and what you can do about them.

In this section, we explore physical and verbal sexual pressures and what to do about each kind.

Resisting Physical Sexual Pressure

Parents encourage their daughters to be on the lookout for strangers and strange places—places where they may be prey to men who wish to take advantage of them. The threat of rape from strangers in strange places is real enough. According to the Bureau of Justice Statistics' National Crime Survey, approximately 70,000 cases of rape were reported to authorities in 1990.[7] It is been estimated that only one rape in five is reported, however. As many as 350,000 rapes may have taken place in 1990.

But stranger rape—as frightening and harmful as it is—largely misses the mark, especially for students who are living away at college. First of all, only about 20 percent of rapes are committed by strangers.[8] Most rapes are committed by people who are well-known to the victim. Many

times they are committed by her dates.

Thousands—perhaps millions—of college women have been victimized by college men, and there is much controversy as to where the lines between rape and 'normal' sexual pressure are to be drawn. Nine percent of a recent sample of over 6,000 college women reported that they had given in to sexual intercourse as a result of threats or physical force.[9] Consider the case of Ann:

> I first met him at a party. He was really good looking and he had a great smile. I wanted to meet him but I wasn't sure how. I didn't want to appear too forward. Then he came over and introduced himself. We talked and found we had a lot in common. I really liked him. When he asked me over to his place for a drink, I thought it would be OK. He was such a good listener, and I wanted him to ask me out again.
>
> When we got to his room, the only place to sit was on the bed. I didn't want him to get the wrong idea, but what else could I do? We talked for a while and then he made his move. I was so startled. He started by kissing. I really liked him so the kissing was nice. But then he pushed me down on the bed. I tried to get up and I told him to stop. He was so much bigger and stronger. I got scared and I started to cry. I froze and he raped me.
>
> It took only a couple of minutes and it was terrible, he was so rough. When it was over he kept asking me what was wrong, like he didn't know. He had just forced himself on me and he thought that was OK. He drove me home and said he wanted to see me again. I'm so

afraid to see him. I never thought it would happen to me.[10]

Forced intercourse is a clear example of rape. The numbers of college women who are subjected to coerced kissing and petting are truly startling, however. Nearly 70 percent of the 282 women in another college sample had been assaulted (usually by dates and friends) at some time since entering college.[11] Of 201 college men surveyed at a major university, 40 percent admitted using coercion to unfasten a woman's clothing, and 13 percent reported that they had forced a woman to engage in sexual intercourse.[12] Forty-four percent of the college women in another study reported that they had 'given in to sex play' because of a 'man's continual arguments and pressure.'[13]

Why Do Men Rape Women? Why do men force women into sex? Sexual pleasure and release are obvious reasons, but they are not the only ones. Rape is also a man's way of expressing social dominance over women or anger toward them.[14]

Many social critics contend that American culture socializes men—including college men—into becoming rapists.[15] Men are generally rewarded for aggressive, competitive behavior. The date rapist could be said to be asserting culturally expected dominance over women. Sexually coercive college males, as a group, also believe that aggression is a legitimate means of getting what they want.[16]

The lessons learned in competitive sports may particularly predispose college men to sexual violence.[17] Coaches often emphasize winning at all costs. College men are taught to vanquish their opponents, even when winning requires injuring or 'taking out' one's opponent. This philosophy may be translated into relationships with women, because college athletes commit a disproportionate number of rapes.[18] Some are gang rapes that are committed by groups of athletes who reside together and 'bond' so powerfully that they share even their sexual experiences.

Sex and sports are united through common jargon. After a date, a college man's friends may ask him, 'Did you score?' or 'Did you get it in?' Note the aggressive competitiveness with which one college man views dating relationships:

> A man is supposed to view a date with a woman as a premeditated scheme for getting the most sex out of her. Everything he does, he judges in terms of one criterion—'getting laid.' He's supposed to constantly pressure her to see how far he can get. She is his adversary, his opponent in a battle, and he begins to view her as a prize, an object, not a person. While she's dreaming about love, he's thinking about how to conquer her.[19]

College men on dates often see their dates' protests as part of a sexual game or contest. One college man said 'Hell, no' when asked whether a particular date had consented to sex. He went on to say, '. . . but she didn't say no, so she must have wanted it, too. . . . It's the way it works.'[20] Jim, the man who raped Ann, said:

> I first met her at a party. She looked really hot, wearing a sexy dress that showed off her great body. We started talking right away. I knew that she liked me by the way she kept smiling and touching my arm while she was speaking. She seemed pretty relaxed so I asked her back to my place for a drink. . . . When she said yes, I knew that I was going to be lucky!
>
> When we got to my place, we sat on the bed kissing. At first, everything was great. Then, when I started to lay her down on the bed, she started twisting and saying she didn't want to. Most women don't like to appear too easy, so I knew that she was just going through the motions. When she stopped struggling, I knew that she would have to throw in some tears before we did it.

She was still very upset afterwards, and I just don't understand it! If she didn't want to have sex, why did she come back to the room with me? You could tell by the way she dressed and acted that she was no virgin, so why she had to put up such a big struggle I don't know.[21]

Women like Ann, on the other hand, may be socialized into becoming victims. The stereotypical feminine role encourages passivity, nurturance, warmth, and cooperation. Women are often taught to sacrifice for their families and not to raise their voices. A woman may thus be totally unprepared to cope with an aggressive man. She may not know what to do and believe that violent resistance is inappropriate for women.

Rape Myths: Do You Harbor Beliefs That Encourage Rape? Many people, including professionals who work with rapists and victims, believe a number of myths about rape, and these myths tend to blame the victim, not the aggressor. For example, a majority of Americans aged 50 and above believe that the woman is partly responsible for being raped if she dresses provocatively.[22] The majority of Americans believe that some women like to be talked into having sex.

Other myths include the notions that 'Only bad girls get raped,' 'Any healthy woman can resist a rapist if she wants to,' and 'Women only cry rape when they've been jilted or have something to cover up.'[23] These myths deny the impact of the assault and transfer blame onto the victim. They contribute to a social climate that is too often lenient toward rapists and unsympathetic toward victims. You may complete the questionnaire on cultural myths and rape on page 74 if you want to learn whether you hold some of the more common myths.

Rape Prevention

Don't accept rides from strange men—and remember that all men are strange.
—Robin Morgan

Given the incidence of stranger rape, it is useful to be aware of things that can be done to prevent it:[24]

- Establish signals and arrangements with other women in an apartment building or neighborhood.
- List only first initials in the telephone directory or on the mailbox.
- Use dead-bolt locks.
- Keep windows locked and obtain iron grids for first-floor windows.
- Keep entrances and doorways brightly lit.
- Have keys ready for the front door or the car.
- Do not walk alone in the dark.
- Avoid deserted areas.
- Never allow a strange man into your apartment or home without checking his credentials.
- Drive with the car windows up and the door locked.
- Check the rear seat of the car before entering it.
- Avoid living in an unsafe building. (When given this piece of advice, college women often protest that their financial mean and housing are limited, so they have to take what they can get. Even so, there are often choices. Women are advised at the very least to make inquiries as to which neighborhoods and buildings are relatively safe.)

Questionnaire—
Cultural Myths that Create a Climate that Supports Rape

The following statements are based on a questionnaire that was constructed by Martha Burt.[25] Read each statement and indicate whether you believe it to be true or false by circling the True or the False. The key is at the bottom of the questionnaire.

True False 1. A woman who goes to the home or apartment of a man on their first date implies that she is willing to have sex.

True False 2. Any woman can get raped.

True False 3. One reason that women falsely report a rape is that they frequently have a need to call attention to themselves.

True False 4. Any healthy woman can successfully resist a rapist if she really wants to.

True False 5. When women go around braless or wearing short skirts and tight tops, they are just asking for trouble.

True False 6. In the majority of rapes, the victim is promiscuous or has a bad reputation.

True False 7. If a girl engages in necking or petting and she lets things get out of hand, it is her own fault if her partner forces sex on her.

True False 8. Women who get raped while hitchhiking get what they deserve.

True False 9. A woman who is stuck-up and thinks she is too good to talk to guys on the street deserves to be taught a lesson.

True False 10. Many women have an unconscious wish to be raped, and may then unconsciously set up a situation in which they are likely to be attacked.

True False 11. If a woman gets drunk at a party and has intercourse with a man she's just met there, she should be considered 'fair game' to other males at the party who want to have sex with her too, whether she wants to or not.

True False 12. Many women who report a rape are lying because they are angry and want to get back at the man they accuse.

True False 13. Many, if not most, rapes are merely invented by women who discovered they were pregnant and wanted to protect their reputation.

■**Answer Key for Questionnaire on 'Cultural Myths that Create a Climate that Supports Rape'** Each item, with the exception of number 2, represents a cultural myth that supports rape. These myths tend to view sex an adversarial game. They stereotype women as flirtatious and deceitful, and tend to blame the victim for whatever happens to her. ■

- Do not pick up hitchhikers, including women, who may be recruiting victims for male companions. This piece of advice may sound paranoid, but we wouldn't be mentioning it unless it had happened.
- Do not talk to strange men in the street.
- Shout 'Fire!' not 'Rape!' People crowd around fires but avoid scenes of violence.

The following tactics may help prevent *date rape:*[26]

- Date in a group. Avoid getting into secluded situations until you know your date very well. (Some men interpret a date's willingness to accompany them to their room as an agreement to engage in sexual activity.)
- Be wary when a date attempts to control you in any way, such as frightening you by driving rapidly or taking you some place you would rather not go.
- Be very assertive and clear concerning your sexual intentions and limits. Women need to be forceful and clear in their communications, spoken and nonverbal.[27] Some rapists, particularly date rapists, tend to misinterpret women's wishes. If their dates begin to implore them to stop during kissing or petting, they construe pleading as 'female gameplaying.' So if kissing or petting is leading where you don't want it to go, be assertive and speak up. The questionnaire on assertiveness on page 77 will give you insight as to where you stand in relation to other college students.
- Stay sober. Many college men interpret a woman's getting drunk as assenting to sex. Moreover, many college students get involved sexually with people they would otherwise refuse when they are drunk.

- Encourage your college or university to offer educational programs about date rape. The University of Washington, for example, offers students lectures and seminars on date rape and provides women with escorts to get home. Brown University requires all first-year students to attend orientation sessions on rape.[28] The point here is for men to learn that 'No' means 'No,' despite the widespread belief that some women like to be 'talked into' sex.
- Talk to your date about his attitudes toward women. If you get the feeling that he believes that men are in a war with women, or that women try to 'play games' with men, you may be better off dating someone else.
- You can find out about attitudes by discussing items from the nearby questionnaire with a man you are considering dating. You can say something like, 'You know, my friend's date said that . . . What do you think about it?' It's a good way to find out if he has attitudes that can lead to trouble.
- A message to men: If you ask a woman out on a date and she accepts, it is not the same thing as consenting to kissing, petting, or sexual intercourse. Even if she asks you out on the date, it is not the same thing as consenting to kissing, petting, or sexual intercourse. Even if she accompanies you to your room or apartment, it is not the same thing as consenting to kissing, petting, or sexual intercourse. Even if she engages in kissing and petting with you, it is not the same thing as consenting to sexual intercourse. The point is this: If a woman says no, you are obligated to take no for an answer.

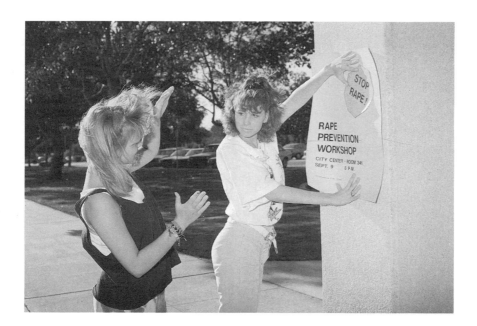

Rape on Campus. *The incidence of rape—including date rape—has reached alarming proportions on campus. Many college women are educating themselves to learn how to protect themselves. Many campuses are also running seminars that educate college men as to where the passionate expression of sexual desire ends and rape begins.*

Resisting Verbal Sexual Pressure

Verbal sexual coercion involves persistent verbal pressure or the use of seduction 'lines' that aim to manipulate another person into sexual activity. Forty-two percent of the respondents to a survey of college men at a southeastern university admitted to verbally coercing a woman into sex.[29] About one in five of the men surveyed at a northwestern university reported having said things to women they did not mean in order to have sexual intercourse.[30] College women in the survey were more likely than men to have been pressured, threatened, or forced into sexual relations. One in four of the women respondents reported that they had sexual intercourse with someone they didn't want to because they had 'felt pressured by his continual arguments.'[31]

Questionnaire—
The Rathus Assertiveness Schedule[32]

Resisting date rape and verbal sexual pressure can mean being assertive—that is, saying what is on your mind clearly and emphatically.

How assertive are you? Do you stick up for your rights, or do you allow others to walk all over you? Do you say what you feel or what you think other people want you to say? When someone tries to pressure you into something you do not want to do, do you say no loudly and clearly, or do you hem and haw and eventually give in?

One way to gain insight into how assertive you are is to take the following self-report test of assertive behavior. You can compare your responses to those of other college students by checking the key on page 81. If you feel that you are too unassertive, why not start to speak up? If you are not sure how to go about it, why not see a counselor at your college counseling center? Many colleges and universities offer training and workshops in assertiveness. Stand up! Speak up! Be yourself!

■ *Directions:* Indicate how well each item describes you by using this code:

+3 = very much like me
+2 = rather like me
+1 = slightly like me
−1 = slightly unlike me
−2 = rather unlike me
−3 = very much unlike me

____ 1. Most people seem to be more aggressive and assertive than I am.*

____ 2. I have hesitated to make or accept dates because of 'shyness.'*

____ 3. When the food served at a restaurant is not done to my satisfaction, I complain about it to the waiter or waitress.

____ 4. I am careful to avoid hurting other people's feelings, even when I feel that I have been injured.*

____ 5. If a salesperson has gone to considerable trouble to show me merchandise that is not quite suitable, I have a difficult time saying 'No.'*

____ 6. When I am asked to do something, I insist upon knowing why.

____ 7. There are times when I look for a good, vigorous argument.

____ 8. I strive to get ahead as well as most people in my position.

____ 9. To be honest, people often take advantage of me.*

____ 10. I enjoy starting conversations with new acquaintances and strangers.

____ 11. I often don't know what to say to attractive persons of the opposite sex.*

____ 12. I will hesitate to make phone calls to business establishments and institutions.*

____ 13. I would rather apply for a job or for admission to a college by writing letters than by going through with personal interviews.*

____ 14. I find it embarrassing to return merchandise.*

____ 15. If a close and respected relative were annoying me, I would smother my feelings rather than express my annoyance.*

____ 16. I have avoided asking questions for fear of sounding stupid.*

____ 17. During an argument I am sometimes afraid that I will get so upset that I will shake all over.*

____ 18. If a famed and respected lecturer makes a comment which I think is incorrect, I will have the audience hear my point of view as well.

____ 19. I avoid arguing over prices with clerks and salespeople.*

____ 20. When I have done something important or worthwhile, I manage to let others know about it.

____ 21. I am open and frank about my feelings.

(continued)

___ 22. If someone has been spreading false and bad stories about me, I see him or her as soon as possible and 'have a talk' about it.

___ 23. I often have a hard time saying 'No.'*

___ 24. I tend to bottle up my emotions rather than make a scene.*

___ 25. I complain about poor service in a restaurant and elsewhere.

___ 26. When I am given a compliment, I sometimes just don't know what to say.*

___ 27. If a couple near me in a theater or at a lecture were conversing rather loudly, I would ask them to be quiet or to take their conversation elsewhere.

___ 28. Anyone attempting to push ahead of me in a line is in for a good battle.

___ 29. I am quick to express an opinion.

___ 30. There are times when I just can't say anything.*

Note this, however: college *men* are also verbally pressured into sexual activity. About one in 15 of the men at the northwestern university admitted having engaged in sexual intercourse against their preferences as a result of sexual pressure. In another study, nearly two out of three college men reported they had been pressured into unwanted sexual intercourse at one time or another.[33] In most cases, sexual pressure took the form of peer pressure or verbal pressure, but in some cases the men reported they were subjected to overt physical coercion.

The use of verbal pressure and 'seduction lines' is very common. Consider the man who deceives a woman into believing that he loves her to persuade her to engage in sexual intercourse. (Saying 'I love you' is not considered a coercive tactic or seduction line when it is sincere, even if it does encourage one's partner to engage in sexual activity.)

Following are some sexual pressure lines and examples of replies that may help you resist them:[34]

KIND OF PRESSURE LINE	THE LINE	SAMPLE RESPONSE
Lines that reassure you about the negative consequences	'Don't worry, I'm sterile.' (Even if the claim is true, sterility offers no protection against H.I.V. and other pathogens.)	'I know you want to make me feel safer, but . . . well, I'm just not comfortable about sex without a condom. I've known a few people who were more fertile than they thought.'
	'You can't get pregnant the first time.' (Untrue, of course. You can also be infected with H.I.V. the first time.)	'Hey, where did you get your sex education? People can get pregnant any time they have intercourse, even if it's just for one second.'

Kind of Pressure Line	The Line	Sample Response
	'Don't worry—I'll pull out.' (Withdrawal before ejaculation will not prevent pregnancy, because some semen can leak out earlier. That semen can also be infected with H.I.V., of course)	'I know you want to reassure me, but people can get pregnant that way, even without ejaculating.'
Lines that threaten you with rejection	'If you don't have sex, I'll find someone who will.'	'I can't believe you are making a threat like this. I'm furious that you would treat lovemaking like some kind of job, as if anyone will do.'
Lines that attempt to put down the refuser	'You're such a bitch.'	'I can't believe you want to make love to me and think calling me names will put me in the mood. Good-bye.'
	'Are you frigid?'	'I resent being called names just because I tell you what I want to do with my body.'
Lines that stress the beautiful experience being missed	'Our relationship will grow stronger.'	'I know you really would like to get more involved right now. But I need to wait. And lots of people have had their relationship grow stronger without intercourse.'
Lines that might settle for less	'I don't want to do anything. I just want to lie next to you.'	'The way we're attracted to each other, I don't think that would be a good idea. As much as I care about you, I'd better not spend the night.'
Lines to make you prove yourself	'If you loved me, you would.'	'You know I care a lot about you. But I feel very pressured when you try to get me to do something I'm not ready for. It's not fair to me. Please consider my feelings.'

KIND OF PRESSURE LINE	THE LINE	SAMPLE RESPONSE
Lines that attempt to be logical, but aren't	'You're my girlfriend—it's your obligation.'	'If you think sex is an obligation, we need to think about this relationship right now.' (*Watch out* for any such talk—it is very common in abusers and rapists. At best, it's an irrational comment by an immature person.)
Lines that are totally transparent	'I'll say I love you after we do it.'	'Bye, now.' (There is no way to deal with a person who would say such a thing.)

Although these sample responses can help you resist specific pressure lines, do not think that 'saying no' to sexual pressure is a privilege that you earn by outarguing your partner. You have the basic right to control your body:

> Some people believe that to resist sexual pressure you have to come up with reasons. So it follows, if your partner gives a good reason, you'd better have a good answer for every reason. Or else. Suppose you are not a very wordy person and you're out with someone who puts a lot of verbal pressure on you. You don't have to engage in a debate! *You don't have to say anything except 'I don't want to.'* It's your body. It's not as if he's asking you to lend him an object that you own. Your body is not an object.[35]

Remember, it's your right to determine how, when, where, and with whom you will share a sexual experience. You may think it is appropriate to offer an explanation in a particular situation, but you do not *have* to explain. Your right to your own body is not debatable.

Sex in this—the age of AIDS—can be risky, but there are a number of things that are as true today as they were in years past. One of them is simply this: AIDS has become just one more reason to make sure that you are ready for sex before becoming involved with sex. When you are not sure about going ahead with sex—because you are not sure about a relationship, because you have concerns about pregnancy, or because you have fears of AIDS and other STDs, there is no harm in waiting. When your partner will not respect your decision to think things through, consider finding another partner. When your partner tells you that other people are more willing and threatens to abandon you for someone who is more willing, you may want to let her or him go. You may be gaining more than you are losing by waiting for someone who will be more understanding about your feelings.

Although sex is important, it is just one part of life. Do you really want to get involved with, or to form a lasting relationship with, someone who is not responsive to your concerns and feelings?

**AIDS Toll-Free Hotline Number:
1-800-342-AIDS**

Scoring Key for the Rathus Assertiveness Schedule. Tabulate your score as follows: For those items followed by an asterisk (*), change the signs (plus to minus; minus to plus). For example, if the response to an asterisked item was +2, place a minus sign (−) before the 2. If the response to an asterisked item was −3, change the minus sign to a plus sign (+) by adding a vertical stroke. Then add up the scores of the 30 items.

Scores on the assertiveness schedule can vary from +90 to −90. The table below will show you how your score compares to those of 764 college women and 637 men from 35 campuses across the United States. For example, if you are a woman and your score was 26, it exceeded that of 80 percent of the women in the sample. A score of 15 for a male exceeds that of 55–60 percent of the men in the sample.

Table 6.1
PERCENTILES FOR SCORES ON THE RAS[36]

Women's Scores	Percentile	Men's Scores
55	99	65
48	97	54
45	95	48
37	90	40
31	85	33
26	80	30
23	75	26
19	70	24
17	65	19
14	60	17
11	55	15
8	50	11
6	45	8
2	40	6
−1	35	3
−4	30	1
−8	25	−3
−13	20	−7
−17	15	−11
−24	10	−15
−34	5	−24
−39	3	−30
−48	1	−41

Notes

Chapter 1

1. Gayle et al. (1990).
2. Altman. (1991, June 18).
3. Suro. (1992, February 19).
4. Osterhout, Formichella, & McIntyre (1991).
5. Specter. (1991, November 9).
6. Johnson. (1990, March 8).
7. Kolata. (1991, November 8).

Chapter 2

1. Shilts. 1988, p. xxi.
2. Wachter. 1992, p. 128.
3. Fogle. (1991).

Chapter 3

1. Cited in Parsons. (1991, November 18), p. A14.
2. Stephens. (1991).
3. Leary. (1992, March 3).
4. Fletcher, et al. (1991).

Chapter 4

1. Osterhout et al., 1991, p. 147.
2. Rhoden. (1992, April 9).
3. Eckholm. (1991, November 17).
4. Ibid.
5. Cable News Network. (1991, July).
6. Goodgame. (1990).
7. Ibid.
8. Holmes, & Kreiss. (1988); Perlez. (1991, March 2).
9. Castro et al. (1988).
10. Bloor, McKeganey, & Barnard. (1990); Plant, Plant, & Thomas. (1990); Waldorf et al. (1990).

11. Grossman. (1991, December 22, p. 46.)
12. Cochran & Mays. (1990).
13. Eckholm, 1991; Jacobsen, Perry, & Hirsch. (1990).
14. But not always. For example, infected mothers may transmit H.I.V. antibodies to their fetuses, but not the virus itself.
15. Osterhout et al., 1991, pp. 145–147.
16. In a 'false positive' test result, a person who is not infected with H.I.V. is falsely reported to be infected. The Western blot test is often used to confirm positive results since ELISA does report a small number of false positive results.
17. Cited on Cable News Network, 1991.
18. McKinney et al. (1991).
19. Graham et al. (1992); McCutchan, (1990); Volberding et al. (1990).
20. Moore, Hidalgo, Sugland, & Chaisson. (1991).
21. Leary, 1992.

Chapter 5

1. Gayle et al., 1990.
2. Boston Women's Health Book Collective. (1984).
3. Mirotznik, Shapiro, Steinhart, & Gillepsie. (1987).
4. Blakeslee. (1992, January 22).
5. Ibid.

Chapter 6

1. Carroll, (1988).
2. DeBuono, Zinner, Daamen, & McCormack. (1990).
3. Johnson, 1990.
4. Hernandez & Smith. (1990).

5. MacDonald, Wells, Fisher, Warren, King, Doherty, & Bowie. (1990).
6. Cowley & Hager. (1991, December 9).
7. Bureau of Justice Statistics. (1991).
8. Gibbs. (1991, June 3).
9. Koss, Gidycz, & Wisniewski. (1987).
10. Trenton State College. (1991, Spring).
11. Kanin & Parcell. (1977).
12. Rapaport & Burkhart. (1984).
13. Koss et al., 1987.
14. Ellis. (1991); Malamuth, Sockloskie, Koss, & Tanaka. (1991).
15. Malamuth et al., 1991; Prentky & Knight. (1991).
16. Rapaport & Burkhart, 1984.
17. Myriam Miedzian, cited in Levy. (1991, September 16).
18. Eskenazi. (1990, June 3).
19. Powell, 1991, p. 55.
20. Celis. (1991, January 2).
21. Trenton State College, 1991.
22. Gibbs, 1991, p. 51.
23. Burt. (1980).
24. Ibid.
25. Boston Women's Health Book Collective, 1984.
26. Rathus & Fichner-Rathus. (1991).
27. Volchko, cited in Celis. (1991, January 2).
28. Celis, 1991.
29. Rathus. (1973).
30. Craig, Kalichman, & Follingstad. (1989).
31. Lane & Gwartney-Gibbs. (1985).
32. Ibid, p. 56.
33. Muehlenhard & Falcon. (1990).
34. Powell, 1991.
35. Ibid., p. 72.
36. Nevid & Rathus. (1978).

Bibliography

Adler, J., et al. (1991, November 18). Living with the virus: When—and how—HIV turns into AIDS. *Newsweek*, pp. 33–34.

Altman, L. K. (1989, April 24). Experts on AIDS, citing new data, push for testing. *The New York Times*, pp. A1, B8.

Altman, L. K. (1991, June 18). W.H.O. says 40 million will be infected with AIDS virus by 2000. *The New York Times*, p. C3.

American Medical Association (1991). AIDS vaccines inch closer to useful existence. *Journal of the American Medical Association, 265*, 1356.

America's Black Forum. (1991, November 24). Group W Video Services, Wash. Produced by Uniworld Inc.

Antoni, M. H., et al. (1990). Psychoneuroimmunology and HIV-1. *Journal of Consulting and Clinical Psychology, 58*, 38–49.

Antoni, M. H., et al. (1991). Cognitive-behavioral stress management intervention buffers distress responses and immunologic changes following notification of HIV-1 seropositivity. *Journal of Consulting and Clinical Psychology, 59*, 906–915.

Barbaree, H. E., & Marshall, W. L., (1991). The role of male sexual arousal in rape: Six models. *Journal of Consulting and Clinical Psychology, 59*, 621–630.

Blakeslee, S. (1992, January 22). An epidemic of genital warts raises concern but not alarm. *The New York Times*, p. C12.

Bloor, M., McKeganey, N., & Barnard, M. (1990). An ethnographic study of HIV-related risk practices among Glasgow rent boys and their clients:

Report of a pilot study. *AIDS Care, 2*, 17–24.

Boston Women's Health Book Collective. (1984). *The new our bodies, ourselves.* New York: Simon and Schuster.

Braude, A. I., Davis, C. E., & Fierer, J. (Eds.) (1986). *Infectious diseases and medical microbiology*, 2nd ed. Philadelphia: W. B. Saunders.

Breiman, K. (1991, February 6). Recording of debate over plan to distribute condoms in New York City public schools. Department of Education, Brooklyn, NY.

Briselden, A. M., & Hillier, S. L. (1990). Longitudinal study of the biotypes of Gardnerella vaginalis. *Journal of Clinical Microbiology, 28*, 2761–2764.

Brock, B. V., Selke, S., Benedetti, J., Douglas, J. M., Jr., & Corey, L. (1990). Frequency of asymptomatic shedding of herpes simplex virus in women with genital herpes. *Journal of the American Medical Association, 263*, 418–420.

Brown, Z. A., et al. (1991). Neonatal herpes simplex virus infection in relation to asymptomatic maternal infection at the time of labor. *The New England Journal of Medicine, 324*, 1247–1252.

Bruce, K. E. M., & Bullins, C. G. (1989). Students' attitudes and knowledge about genital herpes. *Journal of Sex Education and Therapy, 15*, 257–270.

Bureau of Justice Statistics. (1991). *National crime survey.* Washington, D.C.: Government Printing Office.

Burke, D. S., et al. (1988). Measurement of the false positive rate in a screening program for Human Immunodeficiency Virus infections. *The New England Journal of Medicine, 319*, 961–964.

Burt, M. R. (1980). Cultural myths

and supports for rape. *Journal of Personality and Social Psychology, 38*, 217–230.

Busch, M. P., et al. (1991). Evaluation of screened blood donations for HIV-1 infection by culture and DNA amplification of pooled cells. *The New England Journal of Medicine, 325*, 1–5.

Cable News Network. (1991, July). *AIDS issues: Policy for health care providers.* Blackline Master I Segments, 1, 2, 5, 9, 10.

Calderone, M. S., & Johnson, E. W. (1989). *Family book about sexuality*, rev. ed. New York: Harper & Row.

Campbell, C. E., & Herten, R. J. (1981). VD to STD: Redefining venereal disease. *American Journal of Nursing, 81*, 1629–1635.

Carroll, L. (1988). Concern with AIDS and the sexual behavior of college students. *Journal of Marriage and the Family, 50*, 405–411.

Castro, K. G., et al. (1988). Transmission of HIV in Belle Glade, Florida: Lessons for other communities in the United States. *Science, 239*, 193–197.

Catania, J. A., et al., (1991). Changes in condom use among homosexual men in San Francisco. *Health Psychology, 10*, 190–199.

Celis, W. (1991, January 2). Students trying to draw line between sex and an assault. *The New York Times*, pp. 1, B8.

Centers for Diseases Control. (1985). Chlamydia trachomatis infections. *Morbidity and Mortality Weekly Report, 34*, 53.

Centers for Disease Control. (1987). Public Health Service guidelines for counseling and antibody testing to prevent HIV infection and AIDS.

Morbidity and Mortality Weekly Report, *36,* 509–515.

Centers for Disease Control. (1988a) Leads from the MMWR/ Morbidity and Mortality Weekly Report (Vol 37/No.7, 9, 1988). Condoms for prevention of sexually transmitted diseases. *Journal of the American Medical Association, 259,* 1925–1927.

Centers for Disease Control. (1988b). Leads from the MMWR/Morbidity and Mortality Weekly Report (Vol 37, 717–727). HIV-related beliefs, knowledge, and behaviors among high school students. *Journal of the American Medical Association, 260,* 3567, 3570.

Centers for Disease Control. (1988c, April). Prevalence of human immunodeficiency virus antibody in U.S. active military personnel. *Morbidity and Mortality Weekly Report, 37,* 461.

Centers for Disease Control. (1989a). Summaries of identifiable diseases in the United States.

Centers for Disease Control. (1989b). Treatment guidelines for sexually transmitted diseases. *Morbidity and Mortality Weekly Report, 38,* No. S-8.

Centers for Disease Control. (1990). Progress toward achieving the 1990 objectives for the nation for sexually transmitted diseases. *Morbidity and Mortality Weekly Report, 39,* 53–57.

Centers for Disease Control. (1990). Update: Serologic testing for HIV-1 antibody—United States, 1988 and 1989. *Morbidity and Mortality Weekly Report, 39,* 380–383.

Centers for Disease Control. (1990). Estimates of HIV prevalence and projected AIDS cases; Summary of a workshop, October 31–November 1, 1989. *Morbidity and Mortality Weekly Report,* February 23, 110–119.

Centers for Disease Control. (1990). Update: Acquired Immunodeficiency Syndrome—United States, 1989. *Journal of the American Medical Association, 263,* 1191–1192.

Centers for Disease Control. (1990). HIV prevalence estimates and AIDS case projections for the United States: Report based on a workshop. *Morbidity and Mortality Weekly Report, 39,* (No. RR-16), 30.

Centers for Disease Control. (1990). Heterosexual behaviors and factors that influence condom use among patients attending a sexually transmitted disease clinic—San Francisco. *Morbidity and Mortality Weekly Report, 39,* 685–689.

Centers for Disease Control. (1991). AIDS in women—United States. *Journal of the American Medical Association, 265,* 23.

Centers for Disease Control. (1991). Mortality attributable to HIV infection/AIDS—United States, 1981–1990. *Journal of the American Medical Association, 265,* 848.

Centers for Disease Control. (1991). Characteristics of, and HIV infection among, women served by publicly funded HIV counseling and testing services—United States, 1989–1990. *Journal of the American Medical Association, 265,* 2051.

Centers for Disease Control. (1991). Update: Acquired immunodeficiency syndrome—United States, 1991–1990. *Morbidity and Mortality Weekly Report, 40,* 358–369.

Centers for Disease Control. (1991). Summary of notifiable diseases, United States 1990. *Morbidity and Mortality Weekly Report, 39,* 1–53.

Centers for Disease Control (CDC) AIDS Hotline Communications, 1992.

Chu, S. Y., Buehler, J. W., Berkelman, R. L. (1990). Impact of the human immunodeficiency virus epidemic on mortality in women of reproductive age, United States. *Journal of the American Medical Association, 264,* 225–229.

Cochran, S. D. (1988, August). *Risky behavior and disclosure: Is it safe if you ask?* Paper presented at the meeting of the American Psychological Association, Atlanta, GA.

Cochran, S.D., & Mays, V.M. (1989). Women and AIDS-related concerns: Roles for psychologists in helping the worried well. *American Psychologist, 44,* 529–535.

Cochran, S. D. & Mays, V. M. (1990). Sex, lies, and H.I.V. *The New England Journal of Medicine, 322,* 774–775.

Cohen, J. B. (1990, December 13). A crosscutting perspective on the epidemiology of HIV infection in women. Paper presented at the Women and AIDS Conference, Washington, D.C. (abstract).

Craig, M. E., Kalichman, S. C., & Follingstad, D. R. (1989). Verbal coercive sexual behavior among college students. *Archives of Sexual Behavior, 18,* 421–434.

Crum, C., & Ellner, P. (1985). Chlamydia infections: Making the diagnosis. *Contemporary Obstetrics and Gynecology, 25,* 153–159, 163, 165, 168.

Curran, J. W., et al. (1988). Epidemiology of HIV infection and AIDS in the United States. *Science, 239,* 610–616.

Davis, G. L., et al. (1989). Treatment of chronic hepatitis C with recombinant interferon alfa. *The New England Journal of Medicine, 321,* 1501–1506.

DeBuono, B. A., Zinner, S. H., Daamen, M., & McCormack, W. M. (1990). Sexual behavior of college women in 1975, 1986, and 1989. *The New England Journal of Medicine, 322,* 821–825.

DesJarlais, D. C., & Friedman, S. R. (1988). The psychology of preventing AIDS among intravenous drug users: A social learning conceptualization. *American Psychologist, 43,* 865–871.

Eckholm, E. (1991, November 17). Facts of life: More than inspiration is needed to fight AIDS. *The New York Times,* pp. E1, E3.

Ellerbrock, T. V., et al. (1991). Epidemiology of women with AIDS in the United States, 1981 through 1990: A comparison with heterosexual men with AIDS. *Journal of the American Medical Association, 265,* 2971–2975.

Ellis, L. (1991). A synthesized (biosocial) theory of rape. *Journal of Consulting and Clinical Psychology, 59,* 631–642.

Erlanger, S. (1991, July 14). A plague awaits. *The New York Times Magazine,* pp. 24, 26, 49, 53.

Eskenazi, G. (1990, June 3). The male athlete and sexual assault. *The New*

York Times, pp. L1, L4.

Essex, M., & Kanki, P. (1988, October). The origins of the AIDS virus. *Scientific American*, pp. 64–71.

Farley, A. U., Hadler, J. L., & Gunn, R. A. (1990). The syphilis epidemic in Connecticut: Relationship to drug use and prostitution. *Sexually Transmitted Diseases, 17*, 163–168.

Faulstich, M. E. (1987). Psychiatric aspects of AIDS. *American Journal of Psychiatry, 144*, 551–556.

Fischl, M. A., et al. (1990). A randomized controlled trial of a reduced daily dose of zidovudine in patients with acquired immunodeficiency syndrome. *The New England Journal of Medicine, 323*, 1009–1014.

Fletcher, J. M., et al. (1991). Neurobehavioral outcomes in diseases of childhood: Individual change models for pediatric human immunodeficiency viruses. *American Psychologist, 46*, 1267–1277.

Fogle, S. (1991). The advent of AIDS. *The Journal of NIH Research, 3*, 88–91.

Forrest, J. D., & Silverman, J. (1989). What public school teachers teach about preventing pregnancy, AIDS and sexually transmitted diseases. *Family Planning Perspectives, 15*, 65–72.

Fox, M. (1985, December). Interfering with herpes. *Today's Health*, 22.

Fox, R., Odaka, N. J., Brookmeyer, R., & Polk, B. F. (1987). Effect of antibody test disclosure on subsequent sexual activity in homosexual men. *AIDS, 1*, 241–246.

Friedman, S. R., et al. (1987). AIDS and self-organization among intravenous drug users. *International Journal of Addictions, 22*, 201–220.

Friedrich, E. (1985). Vaginitis. *American Journal of Obstetrics and Gynecology, 152*, 247–251.

Garland, S. M., Lees, M. I., & Skurrie, I. J. (1990) Chlamydia trachomatis: Role in tubal infertility. *Australian and New Zealand Journal of Obstetrics and Gynaecology, 30*, 83–86.

Garry, R. F., Witte, M. H., Gottlieb, A. A., Elvin-Lewis, M., Gottlieb, M. S., Witte, C. L., Alexander, S. S., Cole, W. R., & Drake, W. L, Jr. (1988). Documentation of an AIDS virus infection in the United States in 1968. *Journal of the American Medical Association, 260*, 285–287.

Gavey, N. (1991). Sexual victimization prevalence among New Zealand university students. *Journal of Consulting and Clinical Psychology, 59*, 464–466.

Gayle, H. D., et al. (1990). Prevalence of human immunodeficiency virus among university students. *The New England Journal of Medicine, 323*, 1538–1541.

Gibbs, N, (1991, June 3). When is it rape? *Time*, pp. 48–54.

Glasner, P. D., & Kaslow, R. A. (1990). The epidemiology of human immunodeficiency virus infection. *Journal of Consulting and Clinical Psychology, 58*, 13–21.

Goedert, J. J., et al. Cited in Leary, W. E. (1992, January 7). Study of H.I.V. transmission at birth. *The New York Times*, p. C3.

Gold, D., Ashley, R., Solberg, G., Abbo, H., & Corey, L. (1988). Chronic-dose acyclovir, to suppress frequently recurring genital herpes simplex virus infection: Effect on antibody response to herpes simplex virus type 2 proteins. *Journal of Infectious Diseases, 158*, 1227–1234.

Golden, N. (1985). Treating the adolescent with Chlamydia trachomatis infection. *Medical Aspects of Human Sexuality, 19*, 80.

Goldsmith, M. (1986). Sexually transmitted diseases may reverse the 'revolution.' *Journal of the American Medical Association, 255*, 1665–1672.

Goldsmith, M. F. (1987). Sex in the age of AIDS calls for common sense and condom sense. *Journal of the American Medical Association, 255*, 1665–1672.

Goldsmith, M. F. (1989). Medical news and perspectives: 'Silent epidemic' of 'social disease' makes STD experts raise their voices. *Journal of the American Medical Association, 261*, 3509–3510.

Goldsmith, M. F. (1991). Costs in dollars and lives continue to rise. *Journal of the American Medical Association, 266*, 1055.

Goldstein, A. M., & Clark, J. H. (1990). Treatment of uncomplicated gonococcal urethritis with single-dose cefitzoxime. *Sexually Transmitted Diseases, 17*, 181–183.

Goodgame, R. W. (1990). AIDS in Uganda—Clinical and social features. *The New England Journal of Medicine, 323*, 383–389.

Gordon, S., & Snyder, C. W. (1989). *Personal issues in human sexuality: A guidebook for better sexual health*, 2nd ed. Boston: Allyn & Bacon.

Gottlieb, M. S. (1991, June 5). AIDS—the second decade: Leadership is lacking. *The New York Times*, p. A29.

Graham, J. M., & Blanco, J. D. (1990) Chlamydial infections. *Primary Care: Clinics in Office Practice, 17*, 85–93.

Graham, N. M. H., et al. (1992). The effects on survival of early treatment of human immunodeficiency virus infection. *The New England Journal of Medicine, 326*, 1037–1042.

Graham, S., et al. (1982). Sex patterns and herpes simplex virus type 2 in the epidemiology of cancer of the cervix. *American Journal of Epidemiology, 115*, 729–735.

Grossman, S. (1991, December 22). Cited in Undergraduates drink heavily, survey discloses. *The New York Times*, p. 46.

Guinan, M. E. (1992). Cited in Leary, W. E. (1992, February 1). U.S. panel backs approval of first condom for women. *The New York Times*, p. 7.

Gwinn, M. et al. (1991). Prevalence of HIV infection in childbearing women in the United States: Surveillance using newborn blood samples. *Journal of the American Medical Association, 13*, 1704.

Handsfield, H. (1984). Gonorrhea and uncomplicated gonococcal infection. In K. K. Holmes, et al., (Eds.), *Sexually transmitted diseases*. (pp. 205–220). New York: McGraw-Hill.

Handsfield, H. H. (1988). Questions and answers: 'Safe sex' guidelines: Mycoplasma and chlamydia infections.

Journal of the American Medical Association, 259, 2022.

Hardy, A. M., Rauch, K., Echenberg, D., Morgan, W. M., & Curran, J. W. (1986). The economic impact of the first 10,000 cases of acquired immune deficiency syndrome in the United States. *Journal of the American Medical Association, 225,* 209–211.

Harris, R. E., et al. (1990). Changes in AIDS risk behavior among intravenous drug abusers in New York City. *New York State Journal of Medicine, 90,* 123–126.

Hatcher, R. A., et al. (1990). *Contraceptive technology: 1990–1991,* 15th rev. ed. New York: Irvington Publishers.

Heagarty, M. C., & Abrams, E. J. (1992). Caring for HIV-infected women and children. *The New England Journal of Medicine, 326,* 887–888.

Hearst, N., & Hulley, S. B. (1988). Preventing the heterosexual spread of AIDS: Are we giving our patients the best advice? *Journal of the American Medical Association, 259,* 2428–2432.

Hébert, Y., Bernard, J., De Man, A. F., Farrar, D. (1989). Factors related to the use of condoms among French-Canadian university students. *The Journal of Social Psychology, 129,* 707–709.

Hernandez, J. T., & Smith, F. J. (1990). Inconsistencies and misperceptions putting college students at risk of HIV infection. *Journal of Adolescent Health Care, 11,* 295–297.

Hodgson, R., Driscoll, G. L., Dodd, J. K., & Tyler, J. P. (1990). Chlamydia trachomatis: The prevalence, trend and importance in initial infertility management. *Australian and New Zealand Journal of Obstetrics and Gynaecology, 30,* 251–254.

Holmberg, S. D., & Curran, J. W. (1989). The epidmiology of HIV infection in industrialized countries. In K. K. Holmes et al. (Eds.), *Sexually transmitted diseases* (pp. 343–354). New York: McGraw-Hill.

Holmes, K. K., & Kreiss, J. (1988). Heterosexual transmission of human immunodefiency virus: Overview of a neglected aspect of the AIDS epidemic. *Journal of Acquired Immune Deficiency Syndromes, 1,* 602–610.

Holmes, K. K., et al. (1989). (Eds.). *Sexually transmitted diseases,* 2d ed. New York: McGraw-Hill.

Hu, S. (1992, January 24). Cited in Immune deficiency vaccine for monkeys succeeds. *The New York Times,* p. A17.

Imagawa, D. T., et al. (1989). Human immunodeficiency virus type 1 infection in homosexual men who remain seropositive for prolonged periods. *The New England Journal of Medicine, 320,* 1458–1462.

Ison, C. A. (1990). Laboratory methods in genitourinary medicine: Methods of diagnosing gonorrhoea. *Genitourinary Medicine, 66,* 453–459.

Jacobsen, P. B., Perry, S. W., & Hirsch, D. (1990). Behavioral and psychological responses to HIV antibody testing. *Journal of Consulting and Clinical Psychology, 58,* 31–37.

Jenny, C., Hooton, T. M., Bowers, A., Copass, M. K., Krieger, J. N., Hillier, S. L., Kiviat, N., Corey, L., Stamm, W. E., & Holmes, K. K. (1990). Sexually transmitted diseases in victims of rape. *The New England Journal of Medicine, 322,* 713–716.

Johnson, K. (1988). *Teens and AIDS: Opportunities for prevention.* Washington, D.C.: Children's Defense Fund.

Johnson, R. E., et al. (1989). A seroepidemiologic survey of the prevalence of herpes simplex virus type 2 infection in the United States. *The New England Journal of Medicine, 321,* 7–12.

Johnson, D. (1990, March 8). AIDS clamor at colleges muffling older dangers. *The New York Times,* p. A18.

Johnston, L. D., Bachman, J. G., & O'Malley, P. M. (1991, January 23). Monitoring the future: A continuing study of the lifestyles and values of youth. The University of Michigan News and Information Services: Ann Arbor, MI.

Jones, C. C., et al. (1987). Persistence in high risk sexual activity among homosexual men in an area of low incidence of Acquired Immunodeficiency Syndrome. *Sexually Transmitted Diseases, 14,* 79–82.

Jones, D. S., et al. (1992). Epidemiology of transfusion-associated acquired immunodeficiency syndrome in children in the United States, 1981 through 1989. *Pediatrics, 89,* 123–127.

Kagay, M. R. (1991, June 19). Poll finds AIDS causes single people to alter behavior. *The New York Times,* p. C3.

Kanin, E. J., & Parcell, S. R. (1977). Sexual aggression: A second look at the offended female. *Archives of Sexual Behavior, 6,* 67–76.

Kantrowitz, B., et al. (1991, April 29). Naming names. *Newsweek,* pp. 26–32.

Kantrowitz, B., et al. (1991, July 1). Doctors and AIDS. *Newsweek,* pp. 48–57.

Kaplowitz, L. G., et al. (1991). Prolonged continuous acyclovir treatment of normal adults with frequently recurring genital herpes simplex virus infection. *Journal of the American Medical Association, 265,* 747–751.

Kegeles, S., Alan, M. E., & Irwin, C. (1988). Sexually active adoles-cents and condoms: Changes over one year in knowledge, attitudes, and use. *American Journal of Public Health, 78,* 460–461.

Kelly, J. A., Brasfield, T. L., & St. Lawrence, J. S. (1991). Predictors of vulnerability to AIDS risk behavior relapse. *Journal of Consulting and Clinical Psychology, 59,* 163–166.

Kelly, J. A., St. Lawrence, J. S., Hood, H. V., & Brasfield, T. L. (1989). Behavioral intervention to reduce AIDS risk activities. *Journal of Consulting and Clinical Psychology, 57,* 60–67.

Kelly, J. A., & St. Lawrence, J. S. (1988). AIDS prevention and treatment: Psychology's role in the health crisis. *Clinical Psychology Review, 8,* 255–284.

Kemeny, M. E., Cohen, F., Zegans, L. S., & Conant, M. A. (1989). Psychological and immunological predictors of genital herpes recurrence. *Psychosomatic Medicine, 51,* 195–208.

Kent, M. R. (1991). Women and AIDS. *The New England Journal of Medicine, 324,* 1442.

Kiecolt-Glaser, J. K., & Glaser, R. (1988). Psychological influences on immunity: Implications for AIDS. *American Psychologist, 43*, 892–898.

King, W. (1991, December 4). Registry of AIDS-virus carriers is begun. *The New York Times*, p. B3.

Kolata, G. (1991, June 4). 10 years of AIDS battle: Hopes for success dim. *The New York Times*, p. A14.

Kolata, G. (1991, July 20). U.S. panel backs sale of experimental AIDS drug. *The New York Times*, pp. A1, A13.

Kolata, G. (1991, November 8). Studies cite 10.5 years from infection to illness. *The New York Times*, p. B12.

Kolata, G. (1991, November 9). For heterosexuals, diagnosis of AIDS is often mercifully late. *The New York Times*, p. A32.

Kolata, G. (1991, November 28). Theory links AIDS to malaria experiments. *The New York Times*, p. B14.

Koss, M. P., Gidycz, C. A., & Wisniewski, N. (1987). The scope of rape: Incidence and prevalence of sexual aggression and victimization in a national sample of higher education students. *Journal of Consulting and Clinical Psychology, 55*, 162–170.

Kramer, L. (1990, July 16). A 'Manhattan Project' for AIDS. *The New York Times*, p. A15.

Kroger, F. (1991). Cited in Sims, C. (1991, December 7). HIV tests up 60% since the disclosure from Magic Johnson. *The New York Times*, pp. A1, A28.

Lambert, B. (1991, December 9). Kimberly Bergalis is dead at 23; symbol of debate over AIDS tests. *The New York Times*, p. D9.

Landesman, S. H., et al. (1989). HIV disease in reproductive age women: A problem of the present. *Journal of the American Medical Association, 261*, 1326–1327.

Landis, S. E., et al. (1992). Results of a randomized trial of partner notification in cases of HIV infection in North Carolina. *The New England Journal of Medicine, 326*, 101–106.

Lane, K. E., & Gwartney-Gibbs, P. A. (1985). Violence in the context of dating and sex. *Journal of Family Issues, 6*, 45–59.

Laskin, D. (1982, February 21). The herpes syndrome. *The New York Times Magazine*, pp. 94–108.

Leary, W. E. (1992, February 1). U.S. panel backs approval of first condom for women. *The New York Times*, p. A7.

Leary, W. E. (1992, March 3). Progress is reported in cutting AIDS link from mother to child. *The New York Times*, p. C3.

Leishman, K. (1987, February). Heterosexuals and AIDS. *The Atlantic*, pp. 39–58.

Lemp, G. F., Payne, S. F., Neal, D., Temelso, R., & Rutherford, G. W. (1990). Survival trends for patients with AIDS. *Journal of the American Medical Association, 265*, 402.

Levine, G. I. (1991). Sexually transmitted parasitic diseases. *Primary Care: Clinics in Office Practice, 18*, 101–128.

Levy, D. S. (1991, September 16). Why Johnny might grow up violent and sexist. *Time*, pp. 16–19.

Levy, J. A., et al., (1985). Isolation of AIDS-associated retrovirus from cerebrospinal fluid and brains of patients with neurological symptoms. *Lancet, 2*, 586–588.

Levy, M. R., Dignan, M., & Shirreffs, J. H. (1987). *Life & health*, 5th ed. New York: Random House.

Lewin, T. (1991, February 8). Studies on teen-age sex cloud condom debate. *The New York Times*, p. A14.

Lewin, T. (1991, November 29). 5-year contraceptive implant seems headed for wide use. *The New York Times*, p. A1.

Longo, D.J., & Clum, G.A. (1989). Psychosocial factors affecting genital herpes recurrences: Linear vs. mediating models. *Journal of Psychosomatic Research, 33*, 161–166.

Lourea, D., Rila, M., & Taylor, C. (1986). Sex in the age of AIDS. Paper presented to the Western Region Conference of the Society for the Scientific Study of Sex, Scottsdale, AZ.

Lui, K. J., et al. (1988). A model-based estimate of the mean incubation period for AIDS in homosexual men. *Science, 240*, 1333–1335.

MacDonald, N. E., et al. (1990). High-risk STD/HIV behavior among college students. *Journal of the American Medical Association, 263*, 3155–3159.

Malamuth, N. M., Sockloskie, R. J., Koss, M. P., & Tanaka, J. S. (1991). Characteristics of aggressors against women: Testing a model using a national sample of college students. *Journal of Consulting and Clinical Psychology, 59*, 670–681.

Martens, M., & Faro, S. (1989, January). Update on trichomoniasis: Detection and management. *Medical Aspects of Human Sexuality*, 73–79.

Martin, D. H. (1990). Chlamydial infections. *Medical Clinics of North America, 74*, 1367–1387.

Martin, J. L. (1987). The impact of AIDS on gay male sexual behavior pattern in New York City. *American Journal of Public Health, 77*, 578–581.

Martin, J. L. (1988). Psychological consequences of AIDS-related bereavement among gay men. *Journal of Consulting and Clinical Psychology, 56*, 856–862.

Mays, V. M., & Cochran, S. D. (1988). Issues in the perception of AIDS risk and risk reduction activities by Black and Hispanic/Latina women. *American Psychologist, 43*, 499–957.

McCormack, W. M. (1990). Overview. *Sexually Transmitted Diseases, 57*, 187–191.

McCutchan, J. A. (1990). Virology, immunology, and clinical course of HIV infection. *Journal of Consulting and Clinical Psychology, 58*, 5–12.

McKinney, R. E., et al. (1991). A multicenter trial of oral zidovudine in children with advanced human immunodeficiency virus disease. *The New England Journal of Medicine, 324*, 1018–1025.

Melvin, S. Y. (1990). Syphilis: Resurgence of an old disease. *Primary Care: Clinics in Office Practice, 17*, 47–57.

Minkoff, H. L., et al. (1990) The relationship of cocaine use to syphilis and human immunodeficiency virus infections among inner city parturient women. *American Journal of Obstetrics and Gynecology, 163*, 521–526.

Mirotznik, J., Shapiro, R. D., Steinhart, J. E., & Gillespie, O. (1987). Genital herpes: An investigation of its attitudinal and behavioral correlates. *Journal of Sex Research, 23,* 266–272.

Moi, H., et al. (1989). Should male consorts of women with bacterial vaginosis be treated? *Genitourinary Medicine, 65,* 263–268.

Moore, R. D., Hidalgo, J., Sugland, B. W., & Chaisson, R. E. (1991). Zidovudine and the natural history of the acquired immunodeficiency syndrome. *The New England Journal of Medicine, 325,* 1412.

Moran, J. S., & Zenilman, J. M. (1990). Therapy for gonococcal infections: Options in 1989. *Reviews of Infectious Diseases, Suppl. 6.* S633–644.

Muehlenhard, C. L., & Falcon, P. L. (1990). Men's heterosocial skill and attitudes toward women as predictors of verbal sexual coercion and forceful rape. *Sex Roles, 23,* 241–259.

Muehlenhard, C. L., & Linton, M. A. (1987). Date rape and sexual aggression in dating situations: Incidence and risk factors. *Journal of Counseling Psychology, 34,* 186–196.

Navarro, M. (1991, July 23). Women with AIDS virus: Hard choices on motherhood. *The New York Times,* pp. A1, B4.

Navarro, M. (1992, February 10). Agencies hindered in effort to widen definitions of AIDS. *The New York Times,* pp. A1, B11.

Nevid, J. S., & Rathus, S. A. (1978). Multivariate and normative data pertaining to the RAS with a college population. *Behavior Therapy, 9,* 675.

Norman, C. (1986). Politics and science clash on African AIDS. *Science, 230,* 1140–1141.

O'Gorman, E. C., & Bownes, I. T. (1990). Factors influencing behavioural change in response to AIDS educational programmes—the role of cognitive distortions. *Medical Science Research, 18,* 263–264.

Osterhout, M. B., Formichella, A., & McIntyre, S. (1991). *Tell it like it is: Straight talk about sex.* New York: Avon.

Ostrow, D. G., et al. (1989). Disclosure of HIV antibody status: Behavioral and mental health characteristics. *AIDS Education and Prevention, 1,* 1–11.

Parsons, E. (1991, November 18). Women become top U.S. AIDS risk group. *The New York Times,* A14.

Pearson, C. A. (1992). Cited in Leary, W. E. (1992, February 1). U.S. panel backs approval of first condom for women. *The New York Times,* p. A7.

Perlez, J. (1991, March 2). Ugandan wife confronts a custom to avoid AIDS. *The New York Times,* A2.

Perry, S., Jacobsberg, L., & Fogel, K. (1989). Orogenital transmission of human immunodeficiency virus (HIV). *Annals of Internal Medicine, 111,* 951–952.

Peterman, T., Cates, W., & Curran, J. (1988). The challenge of human immunodeficiency virus (HIV) and acquired immunodeficiency syndrome (AIDS) in women and children. *Fertility and Sterility, 49* 571–581.

Plant, M. L., Plant, M. A., Thomas, R. M. (1990). Alcohol, AIDS risks and sex industry clients: Results from a Scottish study. *Drug and Alcohol Dependence, 25,* 51–55.

Platt, R., Rice, P., & McCormack, W. (1983). Risk of acquiring gonorrhea and prevalence of abnormal adnexal findings among women recently exposed to gonorrhea. *Journal of the American Medical Association, 250,* 3205–3209.

Platz-Christensen, J., Larsson, P., Sundstrom, E., & Bondeson, L. (1989). Detection of bacterial vaginosis in Paponicolaou smears. *American Journal of Obstetrics and Gynecology, 160,* 132–133.

Powell, E. (1991). *Talking back to sexual pressure.* Minneapolis: CompCare Publishers.

Prentky, R. A., & Knight, R. A. (1991). Identifying critical dimensions for discriminating among rapists. *Journal of Consulting and Clinical Psychology, 59,* 643–661.

Quinn, T. C. (1990). Unique aspects of human immunodeficiency virus and related viruses in developing countries. In K. K. Holmes, et al. (Eds.), *Sexually transmitted diseases,* 2nd ed. (pp. 355–369). New York: McGraw-Hill.

Quinn, T. C., et al. (1990). The association of syphilis with risk of human immunodeficiency virus infection in patients attending sexually transmitted disease clinics. *Archives of Internal Medicine, 150,* 1297–1302.

Rand, K. H., Hoon, E. F., Massey, J. K., & Johnson, J. H. (1990). *Archives of Internal Medicine, 150,* 1889–1893.

Rando, R. F. (1988). Human papillomavirus: Implications for clinical medicine. *Annals of Internal Medicine, 108,* 628–630.

Ranki, A., et al. (1987). Long latency precedes overt seroconversion in sexually transmitted human immunodeficiency virus infections. *Lancet, 2,* 589–593.

Rapaport, K., & Burkhart, B. R. (1984). Personality and attitudinal characteristics of sexually coercive college males. *Journal of Abnormal Psychology, 93,* 216–221.

Rathus, S. A. (1973). A 30-item schedule for assessing assertive behavior, *Behavior Therapy, 4,* 398–406.

Rathus, S. A., & Fichner-Rathus, L. (1991). *Making the most of college.* Englewood Cliffs, NJ: Prentice Hall.

Rathus, S. A., & Nevid, J. S. (1991). *Abnormal psychology.* Englewood Cliffs, NJ: Prentice Hall.

Redfield, R. R., et al. (1991). A Phase I evaluation of the safety and immunogenicity of vaccination with recombinant gp160 in patients with early human immunodeficiency virus infection. *The New England Journal of Medicine, 24,* 1677–1684.

Reichart, C. A., et al. (1990). Evalution of Abbott Testpack Chlamydia for detection of Chlamydia trachomatis in patients attending sexually transmitted diseases clinics. *Sexually Transmitted Diseases, 17,* 147–151.

Reinisch, J. M. (1990). *The Kinsey Institute new report on sex: What you must know to be sexually literate.* New York: St. Martin's Press.

Reinisch, J. M., Sanders, S. A., &

Ziemba-Davis, M. (1988). The study of sexual behavior in relation to the tranmission of human immunodeficiency virus: Caveats and recommendations. *American Psychologist, 43*, 921–927.

Reuters. (1991, July 10). Clean needles and AIDS. *The New York Times*, p. C11.

Rhoden, W. C. (1992, April 9). An emotional Ashe says that he has AIDS. *The New York Times*, pp. B9, B15.

Richardson, D. (1988). *Women & AIDS*. New York: Routledge, Chapman & Hall.

Rickert, V. I., Jay, M. S., Gottlieb, A., & Bridges, C. (1989). Adolescents and AIDS: Females' attitudes and behaviors toward condom purchase and use. *Journal of Adolescent Health Care, 10*, 313–316.

Riding, A. (1992, Janaury 11). Paris and prostitutes: Withering love. *The New York Times*, p. A4.

Rolfs, R. T., Goldberg, M., & Sharrar, R. G. (1990) Risk factors for syphilis: Cocaine use and prostitution. *American Journal of Public Health, 80*, 853–857.

Rolfs, R. T., & Nakashima, A. K. (1990). Epidemiology of primary and secondary syphilis in the United States: 1981 through 1989. *Journal of the American Medical Association, 264*, 1432–1437.

Rooney, J., Felser, J., Ostrove, J., & Straus, S. (1986). Acquisition of genital herpes from an asymptomatic sexual partner. *The New England Journal of Medicine, 314*, 1561–1564.

Rosenthal, E. (1990, August 28). The spread of AIDS: A mystery unravels. *The New York Times*, pp. C1, C2.

Ruder, A. M., Flam, R., Flatto, D., & Curran, A. S. (1990). AIDS education: Evaluation of school and worksite based presentations. *The New York State Journal of Medicine, 90*, 129–133.

Rundell, J. R., Wise, M. G., & Ursano, R. J. (1986). Three cases of AIDS-related psychiatric disorders. *American Journal of Psychiatry, 143*, 777–778.

Schachter, J. (1989). Why we need a program for the control of *Chlamydia trachomatis*. *The New England Journal of Medicine, 320*, 802–804.

Shafer, M. A., et al. (1989). Urinary leukocyte esterase screening test for asymptomatic chlamydial and gono-coccal infections in males. *Journal of the American Medical Association, 262*, 2562–2566.

Sherman, K. J., et al. (1990). Sexually transmitted diseases and tubal pregnancy. *Sexually Transmitted Diseases, 17*, 115–121.

Shilts, R. (1988). *And the band played on: Politics, people, and the AIDS epidemic*. New York: Penguin Books.

Siegel, K., et al. (1988). Patterns of change in sexual behavior among gay men in New York City. *Archives of Sexual Behavior, 17*, 481–497.

Simonds, R. J., et al. (1992). Transmission of human immunodeficiency virus type 1 from a seronegative organ and tissue donor. *The New England Journal of Medicine, 326*, 726–732.

Simonsen, J. N., et al. (1988). Human immunodeficiency virus infection among men with sexually transmitted diseases: Experience from a center in Africa. *The New England Journal of Medicine, 319*, 274–278.

Sims, C. (1991, December 7). H.I.V. tests up 60% since the disclosure from Magic Johnson. *The New York Times*, pp. A1, A28.

Smith, T. F., et al. (1988). The phylogenetic history of immunodeficiency viruses. *Nature, 33*, 573–575.

Sobel, J. D. (1990). Vaginal infections in adult women. *Medical Clinics of North America, 74*, 1573–1602.

Solkin, C. (1990, November 23). AIDS and the hospital crisis. *New York Perspectives*, p. 13.

Sonenstein, F. L., Pleck, J. H., & Ku, L. C. (1989). Sexual activity, condom use and AIDS awareness among adolescent males. *Family Planning Perspectives, 21*, 152–157.

Sonenstein, F. L., Pleck, J. H., & Ku, L. C. (1990, May). *Patterns of sexual activity among adolescent males*. Paper presented at the Annual Meeting of the Population Association of America, Toronto, Canada.

Spark, R. F. (1991). *Male sexual health: A couple's guide*. Mount Vernon, NY: Consumer Reports Books.

Specter, M. (1991, November 8). Magic's loud message for young black men. *The New York Times*, p. B12.

Specter, M. (1991, November 9). When AIDS taps hero, his 'children' feel pain. *The New York Times*, A1, A32.

Spees, E. R. (1987). College students' sexual attitudes and behaviors, 1974-1985: A review of the literature. *Journal of College Student Personnel, 28*, 135-140.

Sperling, R. S., et al. (1992). A survey of zidovudine use in pregnant women with human immunodeficiency virus infection. *The New England Journal of Medicine, 326*, 857–861.

Spitzer, P. G., & Weiner, N. J. (1989). Transmission of HIV infection from a woman to a man by oral sex. *The New England Journal of Medicine, 320*, 251.

Stephens, T. (1991). AIDS in women reveals health-care deficiencies. *The Journal of NIH Research, 3*, 27–30.

Stephens, T. (1991). AIDS hemophiliacs in tough court battles. *The Journal of NIH Research, 3*, 46–51.

Stermac, L. E., Segal, Z. V., & Gillis, R. (1990). Social and cultural factors in sexual assault. In W. L. Marshall et al. (Eds.), *Handbook of sexual assault: Issues, theories, and treatment of the offender*. New York: Plenum.

Stevenson, R. W. (1991, November 8). Magic Johnson ends his career, saying he has AIDS infection. *The New York Times*, pp. A1, B12.

Stewart, F. H. (1992). Cited in Leary, W. E. (1992, February 1). U.S. panel backs approval of first condom for women. *The New York Times*, p. A7.

Stone, K. M., & Whittington, W. L. (1990). Treatment of genital herpes. *Reviews of Infectious Diseases*, Suppl. 6. S633–644.

Straus, S. E. (1985). Herpes simplex virus infections: Biology, treatment, and prevention. *Annals of Internal Medicine, 103*, 404–419.

Suro, R. (1992, February 19). After weeks of disbelief, Texas town accepts truth: H.I.V. infection in its young. *The New York Times*, p. A12.

Thomason, J. L., & Gelbart, S. M. (1989). Trichomonas vaginalis. *Obstetrics and Gynecology, 74*, 536–541.

Thompson, M. E. (1991). Self-defense against sexual coercion: Theory, research, and practice. In E. Grauerholz and M. A. Koralewski (Eds.), *Sexual coercion: A sourcebook on its nature, causes, and prevention.* (pp. 111–121). Lexington, MA: Lexington Books.

Toomey, K. E., & Barnes, R. C. (1990). Treatment of chlamydia trachomatis genital infection. *Reviews of Infectious Diseases*, Suppl. 6. S645–655.

Touchette, N. (1991). HIV-1 link prompts circumspection of circumcision. *The Journal of NIH Research, 3*, 44–46.

Trenton State College. (1991, Spring). Sexual Assault Victim Education and Support-Unit (SAVES-U) Newsletter.

Tross, S., & Hirsch, D. A. (1988). Psychological distress and neuropsychological complications of HIV infection and AIDS. *American Psychologist, 43*, 929–934.

Turner, C. F., Miller, H. G., & Moses, L. E. (Eds.), *AIDS: Sexual behavior and intravenous drug use.* Washington, D.C.: National Academy Press.

U.S. Department of Health and Human Services, Public Health Service (1986). *Surgeon general's report on acquired immune deficiency syndrome.* Washington, D.C.: Government Printing Office.

Van den Hoek, A., & Van Haastrecht, H. J., & Coutinho, R. A. (1990). Heterosexual behaviour of intravenous drug users in Amsterdam: Implications for the AIDS epidemic. *AIDS, 4*, 449–453.

Van de Perre, P., et al. (1991). Postnatal transmission of human immunodeficiency virus type 1 from mother to infant—a prospective cohort study in Kigali, Rwanda. *The New England Journal of Medicine, 325*,

593–598.

Volberding, P. A., et al. (1990). Zidovudine in asymptomatic human immunodeficiency virus infection. *The New England Journal of Medicine, 322*, 941–949.

Volchko, J. (1991). Cited in Celis, W. (1991, January 2). Students trying to draw line between sex and an assault. *The New York Times*, pp. A1, B8.

Wachter, R. M. (1992). AIDS, activism, and the politics of health. *The New England Journal of Medicine, 326*, 128–133.

Waldorf, D., et al. (1990). Needle sharing among male prostitutes: Preliminary findings of the Prospero Project. *Journal of Drug Issues, 20*, 309–334.

Ward, J. W., et al. (1988). Transmission of human immunodeficiency virus (HIV) by blood transfusions screened as negative for HIV antibody. *The New England Journal of Medicine, 318*, 473–478.

Waugh, M. A. (1990). History of clinical developments in sexually transmitted diseases. In K. K. Holmes, et al. (Eds.), *Sexually transmitted diseases,* 2d ed. (pp. 3–16). New York: McGraw-Hill.

Westrom, L. V. ((1990) Chlamydia trachomatis—clinical significance and strategies of intervention. *Seminars in Dermatology, 9*, 117–125.

Whitley, R., et al. (1991). Predictors of morbidity and mortality in infants with herpes simplex virus infections. *The New England Journal of Medicine, 324*, 450–454.

Winkelstein, W., Jr., et al. (1987). The San Francisco Men's Health Study III. Reduction in human immunodeficiency virus transmission among homosexual/bisexual men. *American Journal of Public Health, 77*, 685–689.

Wolfe, J. L., & Fodor, I. G. (1975). A cognitive/behavioral approach to modifying assertive behavior in women. *The Counseling Psychologist, 5*(4), 45–52.

Wooldridge, W. E. (1991). Syphilis: A new visit from an old enemy. *Postgraduate Medicine, 89*, 199–202.

Yarber, W. L., Torabi, M. R., & Veenker, C. H. (1989). Development of a three-component sexually transmitted diseases attitude scale. *Journal of Sex Education & Therapy, 15*, 36–49.

Yarchoan, R., Mitsuya, H., & Broder, S. (1988). AIDS therapies. *Scientific American, 259*, 110–119.

Zenker, P. N., & Rolfs, R. T. (1990). Treatment of syphilis, 1989. *Reviews of Infectious Diseases*, Suppl. 6. S590–609.

AIDS Toll-Free Hotline Number: 1-800-342-AIDS